Advance Praise for
Getting Back on Your Feet

"I was impressed by the thoroughness with which Sally Pryor covered the topic and was equally impressed by the fact that I was unable to find any other treatise that was anywhere near as comprehensive."
James Garrick, M.D., Center for Sports Medicine, Saint Francis Memorial Hospital

"From a physical therapist's viewpoint, I am pleased to be able to recommend a guide that will help patients help themselves in coping with the difficulties of daily life. Eminently practical, *Getting Back on Your Feet* will be useful to a wide range of mobility-challenged persons."
Catherine Van Olden, Director of Physical Therapy, Rusk Institute of Rehabilitation

"Until this book came along, there was never really a resource that I could refer a patient to. I found *Getting Back on Your Feet* to be an excellent resource for dealing with the difficulties of normal functioning that one must face while undergoing rehabilitation."
Michael Giannone, D.P.M.; Fellow, American College of Foot Surgeons; Diplomate, American Board of Podiatric Surgery; Member, American College of Sports Medicine

". . . a comprehensive and practical approach to the problems of those in wheelchairs and on crutches. To the reader it imparts warmth, motivation, encouragement, and understanding in a fashion that is quite rare in medical literature."
Howard A. Rusk, Jr., President of the World Rehabilitation Fund, Inc.

"*Getting Back on Your Feet* is the answer to the needs for mobility-impaired patients of all kinds—including those with arthritic and neurologic conditions. It provides answers to everyday problems which physical therapists, who often concentrate on other areas of recovery, have little experience with. My future patients will be spared a lot of unnecessary trial and error thanks to *Getting Back on Your Feet*."
Betsy Colhoun, Physical Therapist

Getting Back on Your Feet......................

How to Recover Mobility and Fitness After Injury or Surgery to Your Foot, Leg, Hip, or Knee

Sally R. Pryor Illustrations by Joan E. Thomson

Chelsea Green Publishing Company
Post Mills, Vermont

Chelsea Green Publishing Company
P.O. Box 130, Route 113
Post Mills, VT 05058-0130

Printed and bound in the United States of America
First printing April, 1991

Library of Congress Cataloging-in-Publication Data

Pryor, Sally R., 1932-
    Getting back on your feet: a complete guide to recovering fitness
& mobility after injury or surgery on your ankle, foot, leg, hip, or
knee by Sally R. Pryor
        p. cm.
    Includes bibliographical references and index.
    ISBN 0-930031-38-5 (pbk. : alk. paper): $16.95
    1. Extremities, Lower—Wounds and injuries—Patients—
Rehabilitation. 2. Extremities, Lower—Surgery—Patients—
Rehabilitation. 3. Physical therapy. I. Title.
RD798.P74 1990
617.5'803—dc20   90-28242
                                                               CIP

Acknowledgments

With deep thanks to the following people who have helped with encouragement and advice from the very beginning: Dr. Norman Vincent Peale, Dr. James Garrick, Dr. Robert Waters, Dr. Douglas Clark, Dr. Caroline McCagg, Dr. Michael Giannone, Howard Rusk, Jr., William Oetting, P.T., Catherine Van Olden, P.T., and Betsy Colhoun, P.T.

Additional heartfelt thanks are due to Mark Burgeson, who helped the author develop "computer-ease"; to Stephanie Overholt, P.T., who critiqued the entire manuscript, not once, but several times; and to Prudence Read, whose photographic expertise provided the basis for the illustrations.

Contents

Foreword

Finally, an authoritative guide on crutch ambulation has been written from a patient's perspective. This information is long overdue, since so much of the rehabilitation process is directed towards restoring mobility.

The ability to transport oneself from one place to another is essential for nearly all customary activities of daily living including vocational, recreational, and social pursuits. Crutches—and sometimes other assistive aids—are essential when mobility is limited, and it has always surprised me that so little has been written on this subject. This is more astonishing when one considers that patients who utilize crutches for swing-through gait have a significantly greater energy expenditure than their normal counterparts. Like most athletic endeavors, using crutches requires training and attention to technique to be done properly.

The author describes in very clear and succinct language how to use crutches. Yet, *Getting Back on Your Feet* does much more than that because it addresses the key issues encountered in activities of daily living and suggests realistic, practical solutions to everyday situations encountered by those with impaired mobility. Each chapter provides a logical and concise description of the optimal strategies and techniques to maximize function and increase independence.

Getting Back on Your Feet fills a long neglected void and will be of use to physicians, physical therapists, and other health professionals as well.

The groundwork of rehabilitation aims for reintegration into society. Mobility in the environment is a critical factor in this process. *Getting Back on Your Feet* is an excellent resource which will maximize the potential of a favorable outcome for anyone recovering from lower limb injury or surgery.

Robert L. Waters, M.D.
Medical Director, Rancho Los Amigos Medical Center
Director, Regional Spinal Cord Injury Care System of Southern California

● ●

Caution

Getting Back on Your Feet is intended to provide fundamental information for the mobility-impaired person, as an adjunct to medical and therapeutic treatments. Although the ideas and techniques have worked for many individuals, because of your age, weight, strength, judgment, physical conditioning, or other medical problems, parts of this book may not work for you. If in doubt, consult your physician first.

The exercises presented here should not be considered as a substitute for physical therapy by trained professionals.

The illustrations are to provide an idea of described techniques, but cannot be exact in every detail, due to individual differences in disability, physical strength, or biomechanics.

Getting Back on Your Feet is not meant to substitute for your physician's advice and supervision. When in doubt, ask your health professional and in all circumstances, follow his or her recommendations.

Introduction

Getting Back on Your Feet is a handbook of recovery and fitness for the approximately two million Americans each year who have injuries to—or surgery on—their knees, ankles, feet, hips, and legs. It is intended to spare them the customary "hunt-and-peck" method of learning to manage crutches or other mobility aids, to speed their recovery through approved exercise, to increase their knowledge of fitness and how to maintain it to prevent further injury, and to make it possible to return to work, school, or household and child management in the shortest time possible.

With the enormous proportion of Americans actively involved in injury-producing sports, with the number of high-tech joint reconstructions and replacements increasing every year, and with accidents, as always, producing their share of injury and surgery, more and more of us have found or will find ourselves having to cope quickly and successfully with temporary walking impairment—thrust suddenly from an active and unrestricted life to one where the most normal, taken-for-granted activity becomes immensely difficult, time-consuming, and psychologically defeating. Only those who have experienced it can appreciate the unforgettable shock of losing one's freedom to move as one pleases or the unexpected difficulty of doing anything at all, little or large. Such freedom and ease—snatched away so swiftly—are suddenly precious gifts of a former life.

This guide is about regaining your freedom and ease as quickly as possible, even while you adapt to the restrictions of your injury or surgery. It provides essential information, word-to-the-wise recommendations, subtle tips, categorical precautions, and explicit techniques from basic to advanced, each of which has been employed and refined by people who've had injuries and operations just like yours—people who have learned the hard way, through trial and error, and are sharing their hard-won experience with you.

Getting Back on Your Feet will spare you the fears and frustrations of the "win some, lose some" system of recovery during the coming weeks or months. Better yet, when fears and frustrations are a thing of the past and your recovery allows more daring moves, methods of mastering far-out forms of fun are suggested and encouraged. From beginning to end, *Getting Back on Your Feet* will save you incredible amounts of time and energy while you learn to cope with flair and finesse with any type of knee and ankle, foot, hip, or leg injury.

For the moment, though, it ain't easy. It's quite likely that you are employing an unfamiliar arrangement of wooden sticks to "crutch up" or substitute for an injured leg or foot. Having to use crutches is most people's idea of a nightmare. Only gloriously uninhibited children fly off into the great blue yonder, maneuvering their tiny crutches as if they had been born to it.

Mature folk, you and I, are a different matter. We're bigger—we have farther to fall. We're "wiser"—the consequences of further injury or more pain are all too uppermost in our minds. And unlike the little guys who have us to wait on them, while we recover from injury or an operation we not only have to take care of ourselves, we have to take care of a home and to go to our jobs as well. Doing all this while using crutches or other mobility aids (or simply while favoring a leg) is not easy.

Getting Back on Your Feet is written to help you do almost all those things you normally do, safely and with the least expenditure of energy possible. Safety is essential, of course; but you will also quickly discover that conserving strength is equally essential. Getting around on crutches or any other aid can be very tiring in the best of circumstances. If, in addition, you've just had surgery or have led a fairly sedentary life, the first weeks can be exhausting.

But, take heart. Instead of learning the hard way after weeks of struggling, you have here the know-how to quickly adapt to the difficulties that all leg injuries and operations present. Included are specific techniques to help you become proficient with any of the various mobility aids you may require during progressive stages of recovery. If you're using crutches, *Getting Back on Your Feet* will give you the confidence that leads to independence.

Lastly, *Getting Back on Your Feet* addresses the crucial goal of *preventing* injury—either new injury or reinjury—through a graduated series of total-body exercises combined with informative explanations of some of the modern concepts of exercise and sport, concepts that any person interested in regaining and retaining fitness should be familiar with. Precautions on how to avoid injury are sprinkled throughout, along with suggestions on how to exercise safely while recovering from leg injury. Equipment and other recovery resources are listed in Chapter 19.

Each chapter deals with an area or aspect of daily life that is usually found challenging by the "gimp-and-limp" set. Each chapter is also entirely self-contained, so that you are able to refer to any area freely—without reading in sequence—as soon as you are ready or in need. You will be learning and adopting specific strategies to save energy, to save time, and to become adept and able to pursue as full and varied a recovery as possible. You'll be "up" mentally, you'll have a happier frame of mind, and physically you will be in better shape for the big day when you get off those crutches or are cleared for full activity. Hopefully, *Getting Back on Your Feet* will have enabled you to participate in more activities during recovery than you ever dreamed possible.

> *Caution:* Because of other medical problems, your age, strength, weight, or physical conditioning, parts of this book may not apply to you. When in doubt ask your health professional. In all circumstances, follow your doctor's orders.

1　Positive Imaging in Dealing with Injury, Recovery, and Rehabilitation

One of the unpleasant facts of life is that—in the proverbial blink of an eye—injury or illness can rob anyone of independent mobility and with it his or her sense of confidence and self-esteem. Feelings of frustration, uselessness, and dependence may be overwhelming, and jobs and joys previously taken for granted are jeopardized if not downright impossible.

One's sense of being is tied up with cherished activities, whether work or play, and the more these are prohibited, the harder it is to cope. Some people succumb more readily to such frustrating and trying experiences than others. During this time of unimagined shock—when you find yourself sidelined for weeks or months—it is *ego strength* that must be encouraged and developed: the ability to face the facts of one's situation, and muster the will to prevail. Developing ego strength is an essential first step in the long process of recovery.

Professional athletes and amateur sports addicts alike have an especially difficult time dealing with immobilizing injury. The foundation of their participation in the world, their body, becomes nonfunctional, or imperfectly functional—all of a sudden a trap rather than a temple. Their self-image is battered, and worse yet, uncertainty about their future role has crept in. In the back of their minds is the possibility—or the certainty—of never being the same again. Yet most athletes, professional and otherwise, are exceptionally disciplined and motivated because of the demands of their sport. If you are such a person, this strength of purpose is an incalculable asset in your arsenal of coping strategies and ego strength. Use it and get on with recovery.

Dr. Julius Segal, in *Winning Life's Toughest Battles: The Roots of Human Resilience*, writes that everyone has "undreamed-of powers of healing and growth." Dr. Segal has singled out six "strategies" that tap these powers to help people focus on what can be achieved, rather than what has been lost, either temporarily or permanently.

1. Seize the initiative and take control: Don't sit and sorrow. If you can't do everything, do not refuse to do what you can. Being active and keeping your mind busy do wonders in overriding pain and other problems. Determine to and start to acquire the skills needed for independence and fulfillment, accepting and working with the reality of today.

2. Keep in touch with others: Boredom and self-pity develop when you allow yourself to be separated from persons or events which keep life interesting, which arouse curiosity or enlarge the range of your senses. Your work, hobbies, and other activities that keep you in contact with family, business associates, and friends will add balance and realism to your feelings about your situation.

Unhappily, just when you need them most, friends or coworkers sometimes seem in short supply, even appearing to have abandoned you. It's not a way of saying they never really liked you; more likely they just don't know what to say. Since you've probably been in the position of putting off similar calls yourself, be willing to make the initial contact — and as many more as are necessary.

3. Find meaning and purpose in your situation: "Like tea bags, we don't know our own strength until we get into hot water," Dr. Segal says. Although no one would *choose* adversity, when there is no alternative it can be beneficial to be reminded of all we've taken for granted — to reapproach life with a resolve and with a freshness previously abandoned. The ultimate goal could be an obligation to make one's experience count for something, to nurture something special from it or contribute something special somewhere else.

4. Clear your conscience: Dr. Segal's survivors draw a line between behavior and character. They do not think something bad or disagreeable happened to them because they are the sort of people to whom such things happen.

5. Keep hoping: Plan for the future, and expect that things will improve someday, even if you may not get back to where you were before. Develop as active an attitude toward life as is possible. Challenges and adventures still are out there.

6. Above all, reach out and help someone else: Thinking of others is the best antidote, Dr. Segal feels, for "muting the impulse for self-absorption and self-pity." Here is the time and an opportunity for devotion to a cause or person, to find new ways to put meaning into life. A sense of unselfish accomplishment often generates well-being that spills over to help the process of one's *own* physical and mental recovery.

There is a balance that must be achieved during recovery and rehabilitation—a balance between a sensible awareness of limits imposed by one's injury, and the focused mental attitude necessary to overcome pain and boredom.

A focused mental attitude is a combination of determination and persistence. Such an attitude is of enormous help in developing the "can-deal-with-it" approach needed for boredom and pain—when it hurts to turn the wrong way in sleep, when it hurts to get out of bed in the morning, when it hurts to warm up—when it just *hurts,* period. Luckily, the painful period of most leg injuries or operations is soon over, whereas the tedium of rehabilitation—when one's brain rushes ahead and one's body wallows behind—seems interminable. Nurture that mental toughness, that potent combination of persistence and determination, to help you get through the pain and the boredom.

On the other hand, when active rehabilitation commences, each person must develop a sensitivity to his or her injury and level of tolerance for pain, learning to walk a fine line between prudence and imprudence. From the very beginning you will constantly be called upon to make judgments, to listen to your body, and to take care of it while not babying yourself. If there is swelling in your injured leg, do you stop? How do you draw the line between soreness, which is expected, and pain, which is reason to back off? How do you alleviate the excruciating boredom of repetitive exercise? On "bad" days, when you are especially discouraged, do you force yourself on or do you knock off and have some fun?

One can't consult a doctor or therapist with every uncertainty. Get to know your own body best. Participate in the making of decisions that affect your body. Feeling some mastery over your situation will assist in maintaining equilibrium during this frustrating and stressful period.

Most likely your period of recovery will pass a lot quicker than you think. Researchers have found that time seems to go by more quickly during an extended ordeal. Recovering from knee surgery, a badly sprained ankle, or a torn hamstring *is* an ordeal. The founder of rehabilitation therapy, Dr. Howard Rusk, advises "to reach out and get yourself off your hands." So take control. You'll find kindness and support, encouragement and affection all around you. Use the coping strategies above and the how-to strategies which follow to create an active, independent, and safe recovery.

Taking Control of Your Recovery 2

Coming back from any leg injury is a drag. Regardless of differences between various injuries or operations, or whether your rehabilitation is going to take days, weeks or months, there are ways to make recovery much, much easier, as well as much safer. This book is intended to help you do what you want to do and get you where you want to go—at home, at work, or at play—as quickly as possible. Starting at the very beginning, your physician will probably prescribe some or all parts of the treatment plan known by the mnemonic, "RICE"—which stands for rest, ice, compression, and elevation. Later on, the principles of RICE will be applied to other stages of recovery and are useful to know for any future injury.

"RICE"—REST, ICE, COMPRESSION, ELEVATION

"RICE is nice": a good way to remind yourself how best to reduce swelling (and the pressure-causing pain that accompanies it) immediately after injury and/or surgery. Remember, especially in the case of sprains, that healing can be prolonged by months without immediate cooling, proper compression, and elevation. Rest and elevation sort of go together—agreeably uncomplicated—but see below for more detailed suggestions on RICE in general.

Caution: Check with your doctor first when in doubt about applying the RICE treatments.

Rest

At first rest will mean lying around with your injured leg elevated. Then it will probably mean resting your foot, ankle, knee, or leg by getting around on crutches or some other mobility aid.

7

Ice

Immediate application of ice following injury, to constrict blood vessels in the area of injury, is essential to reduce bleeding and swelling. Swelling is most pronounced during the first 6 hours and, if extreme, can actually interfere with blood flow to the extremity. The ice pack should be covered in a towel and applied directly—or the injured part immersed in the coldest water available, iced if possible. Chipped ice is preferable to cubes for ice packs, because it conforms to the shape of the leg. A cast can have an ice pack—in a waterproof bag—placed right on the location of injury. Application of cold should be limited to 15 minutes, followed by 15–30 minutes without, in alternation for the first 24–36 hours.

● ● ●Word to the Wise: POST-EXERCISE ICING. When use of your injured leg is permitted, icing of the affected area after exercise can be extremely important in reducing inflammation and pain caused by the activity, both now and for a long time to come. Consult your doctor or physical therapist and, above all, do not underestimate the value of post-exercise icing.

Caution: Under most circumstances heat should never be applied immediately after injury, since it promotes bleeding of injured tissue. When swelling is no longer increasing, generally 24–48 hours after injury, warmth is recommended to enhance blood flow and healing. (Ankle rehabilitation often starts with slow-motion flexing, such as describing letters of the alphabet in water with the foot, while soaking the injured ankle in a warm bath.) Also, "contrast baths" may be prescribed, in which heat and ice are alternated.

Compression

Correct compression—done immediately after injury—is crucial, helping your body to reabsorb all the fluid resulting from tissue insult. Compression is used only for hands, wrists, ankles, and feet, because application elsewhere can obstruct circulation. Hollows—particularly in the ankle area—should be surrounded and filled in with horseshoe-shaped padding around both sides of the ankle knobs before strapping with an Ace bandage. Ankle wraps that do not uniformly compress the injured area can increase swelling. (Padding can be improvised from any available material such as toweling, rags, or clothing.) Bandaging should be firm but still allow two fingers to be inserted underneath. Compression anywhere that is too tight interferes with the blood flow necessary for tissue health.

Ice and compression: If done immediately after injury, compression with ice — applied simultaneously on top of the bandage — is now considered three times more effective in controlling swelling than icing and compression done separately.

Elevation

Elevation of a leg, to be effective, requires that the leg be raised above the level of your heart — not just propped on a chair at waist height. Elevation allows gravity to assist in the draining of fluids away from the injury site and is especially important during the first 24 hours following injury or surgery. Think "toes above the nose" — day *and* night. There are different methods:

Lying down: Raising your leg on multiple pillows provides good lift when you are lying down in bed or on the couch. In bed you can also create elevation — without the problem of rolling off pillows when asleep — by placing a small suitcase, a sturdy carton, (or your unused encyclopedias), under the mattress.

Sitting: It is difficult to elevate the leg when sitting, but if you have a bar stool handy to perch the leg on and can manage the awkward position, it is one solution. Placing your bad leg up on a table is another solution — or make do with pillows piled on a regular chair. Best of all, if you have the room and the dollars, would be a mechanical recliner chair.

> *Caution:* With the exception of the recliner chair, sitting for long periods in the positions described should be avoided due to stress on the back. In addition, after the initial period of prescribed elevation, too many hours of "normal" sitting — *without* alternate standing or walking — can promote swelling and retard recovery.

Differences in Weight-Bearing Status

Whether or not you are allowed to place weight on an injured leg depends on what you've done to it — or have had done to it. Generally, some type of assistive device will be prescribed to help you manage proper weight-bearing or non-weight-bearing. Crutches, canes, walkers and wheelchairs are all options; sometimes several of them are used in the various stages of prescribed weight-bearing. Crutches, practical and economical because they can be used in all those stages, are discussed in detail in Chapter 5. Recovering while using a cane, a walker, or a wheelchair, is explored in Chapter 6.

Non-weight-bearing: The injured limb may not support any weight at all, or even come in contact with the ground.

Toe touch: The toes or ball of the foot may be placed on the ground for balance only.

Partial-weight-bearing: Your doctor may restrict you to placing a specific percentage of your weight on the injured limb. If available, step on a set of scales with the injured leg to feel what that percentage (generally 25 percent) feels like.

Weight-bearing to tolerance: On your doctor's orders, this regimen allows normal walking within the limits of acceptable and appropriate pain and swelling. Using a cane at this stage is a wise move, as it promotes normal gait while weak muscles gain strength.

Caution: There is a lot of leeway in the prescription of "weight-bearing to tolerance." Build up slowly or you will end up reinjured or with a new injury. One therapist suggests the following "rules of the road" for increased activity of any kind:

Green light. All systems are tolerant of the activity or exercise. Continue.

Yellow light. There is some discomfort but no worsening of the condition. Proceed with caution.

Red light. The activity is progressively worsening the symptoms. Stop and consult with your doctor or therapist.

COPING WITH A CAST

It's no secret that carrying weight around uses more energy. What affects persons with leg injuries is where that weight is carried. Loads placed on the foot—or your leg—raise energy expenditure tremendously, an excellent reason to beg for the lightest cast possible. (Note that cast time can now be reduced in some cases, particularly leg fractures, by newly developed treatment using ultrasound.)

Caution: If any of the following conditions develop, call your doctor:

1. *Secretions.* Any fluid coming through the cast.

2. *Unusual symptoms.* Unusual pain, tingling and numbness, tightness with loss of feeling, or pain due to the cast's impairing circulation. Keep a sharp eye on your toes — left exposed so you can observe their color as well as test their flexibility. If toes become blue or swollen, dial your doc.

3. *Soreness or irritation of the skin.* These may be caused by rubbing of the cast. The skin should not be allowed to get broken.

4. *Immobile big toe.* Inability to raise the big toe is another sign to call your doctor.

5. *Damage to the cast.* A badly damaged cast cannot do its job and may need replacing.

6. *Looseness.* A loose cast that is causing pain may need replacing.

Cast Problems

Moisture: Keep a plaster cast dry — including the heel — not only when bathing but in the rain. Latex cast protectors are available at medical-supply companies, or you can wear a plastic bag, held in place by a rubber band — placed on the cast, not on your leg. Fiberglass casts do not require as much protection from water damage. See Chapter 10 for suggestions on bathing.

Openings: Do not put objects in cast openings. Itching is often a side effect of healing tissue, but scratching only promotes more itching and the possibility of infection.

Powder: Do not put powder of any kind in cast openings if you have had surgery. If there is no incision, corn starch is sometimes used to alleviate itching and is preferable to talcum powder.

Sharp places: Smooth off sharp places on the outside of the cast, including the heel, with a fine grade of sandpaper. Both your healthy leg — and your floor — will be grateful.

Heel: Do not walk on any cast without a walking heel or cast boot, and wait 48 hours after application before using a walking cast.

Cleaning: To remove unwelcome inscriptions on your cast, or to make room for more, wipe them off with a thoroughly wrung-out damp cloth.

SWELLING AND OTHER DISCOMFORTS

After your cast comes off loss of tissue conditioning can bring about swelling (edema) when you first start reusing your injured leg. Do not be concerned; as your leg muscles get revved up, circulation will improve, and the swelling will disappear. The following tips may also help to control swelling:

Support hose: For long-term walking restrictions check with your doctor about the use of support stockings, which help circulation, control swelling, and enhance comfort.

Avoidance of salt: Salt is thought to promote swelling in the lower extremities. With your doctor's agreement, you may wish to use salt substitutes.

Unexpected Areas of Discomfort—Just So You Know

Coldness of the injured leg: Another consequence of immobility is decreased circulation, resulting in chilling of the foot and leg. If you're in a cast, a pair or two of oversized wool socks will keep your toes comfortable; if there is no cast, leg warmers of the sort worn by dancers or aerobic athletes—alone or over a sock or stocking—are perfect, fitting easily and almost invisibly under men's as well as women's pants—even skirts, if they are long enough. Not elegant, perhaps, but toasty.

Caution: If you have joint or muscle problems in your uninjured leg, do not aggravate them by overuse, twisting, rotating, or any other activity.

Soreness on the injured side: You'll also find that muscles in the buttocks' area on the injured side will complain and act unhappy about holding up their unaccustomed burden. Such pains will disappear as you build up these muscles through use. In the meantime, don't get too ambitious before being certain they will take you to where you want to go—and back.

Problems with the uninjured leg: Once you think about it, it won't surprise you that your "good-side" foot, leg, and thigh muscles, which are your only means of locomotion and support if you are in a non-weight-bearing regimen, start aching from the extra use. The sole of that good foot is especially vulnerable and can become very sore. Inserting a foam or lamb's wool pad in your shoe will help relieve the discomfort; if you have an orthotic device, it can sometimes be adjusted or even padded itself.

Relapses: Healing of injury takes a long time, but when you get back to walking and other former activities, you may mistakenly take for granted that the lengthy rest, recuperation, and rehabilitation have brought all your systems to their peak of fitness. Alas, no matter how faithfully you have been rehabbing, *any* new activity can put unaccustomed stress on the injured area, and a bewildering variety of painful complaints may be experienced for a good while to come. Your foot and ankle, unused for so long, may be quite sore. Do not panic: each interim pain does not signal that the operation was a failure or that the injury will leave you in permanent agony. Give every new activity multiple short tryouts, always expecting some initial discomfort. Such symptoms will probably subside as time passes. Time is the key; at the end of a year you will look back and probably recall a lot of alarming pains that are not a factor anymore — at the end of two years even the recall will be gone.

> *Caution:* When in doubt about any new pain or symptom, check with your doctor.

FOOTWEAR

Your shoes should be flat and rubber-soled if possible, with good support. If you are non-weight-bearing, it is vital that the shoe of your *working* foot have a well-cushioned sole to protect it from the burdens of overuse. It's quite likely you'll need to add a lamb's wool pad, anyway, of the sort commonly found in drugstores and supermarkets.

Shoe for walking with a leg cast: For easier walking and clearance for the casted limb, the shoe on your good side should have a higher and wider heel. A temporary lift of an inch or two can be added to the heel of your everyday, "working" shoe by a shoemaker to solve your leg imbalance.

Women's needs: Men will have no trouble at all with the basic footwear guidelines, but women, who want to retain an "image" of some sort, may be forced to invest in one pair of dressy flats to carry them through this difficult footwear period. If the soles are smooth leather rather than rubber, roughen the "working" sole by scratching it hard with the point of a knife or scissors.

Athletic shoes: Conveniently, with athletic shoes nowadays having both jazzy looks and status, you can wear them just about any time or anywhere — and, to be realistic, your public prefers that you go safely rather than glamorously. You'll soon discover that using mobility aids gives you license for all sorts of courtesies and dispensations; on the other hand, in many areas of living you'll wish there were vastly more consideration of your struggles and needs.

LIFESTYLE CAUTIONS

Many preventable falls occur because of something in the environment, such as a loose rug or poor lighting. Assistive aids make you even more vulnerable to obstacles: do something about such hazards *now*.

Rugs: Get rid of scatter rugs, or any rugs that are not firmly in place, for the duration of your assistive-aid life. Ironically, such rugs are *increasingly* hazardous as you become more confident, more freewheeling — and less wary. Doormats, if necessary, can be tacked down.

Damp, wet surfaces: Watch out for these. Whether it's a slippery kitchen floor, a slimy garage, wet leaves, or an icy sidewalk, your aids must be manipulated with utmost caution. Be especially alert for barely visible films of oil in parking areas and garages or on streets; the slightest touch of moisture on top will make them even more treacherous. Treat all such situations as if you were in your car during the first winter snowstorm — slow, and in lowest gear; take small steps and keep the crutches tucked in close to your body.

Floor joints and seams: Watch out that these do not become sliding tracks for your cane, walker, or crutch tips.

Waxed floors: Avoid waxing — or use nonskid wax — until you have not only graduated from assistive aids, but have resumed normal and stable walking. Waxed floors in the kitchen can be especially dangerous because of spilled liquids. Check crutch, walker, or cane tips for wax buildup.

Steps: Where steps or level changes are poorly lighted, mark them with reflective tape and improve lighting with nightlights or spotlights aimed at the stairs or hazardous area.

Stairs: If handrails are not present, they should be installed where at all possible.

Pets: Loving and rambunctious dogs are the main focus here, although it would be wise to keep your eyes peeled for cats on the loose. The best way to protect yourself from friendly canine greetings is to stabilize yourself against a wall of some sort; if the dog jumps, it won't knock you over, and you will be in a stable position to fend it off.

Always try to have loose dogs where you can see them—outdoors *and* indoors—so they don't bowl you over from behind. It's "dogs first" (not "ladies first") going through doors, and dogs first going up stairs.

If your pooch is overly enthusiastic when you return from a car trip, stay seated and greet and calm the dog down before exiting the vehicle. Then keep your back against the car in case of any leftover emotion.

Alcoholic beverages: Beware! Teetotaling is almost as highly recommended when you are crutching, as when you are behind the wheel of a car. Whether indoors or out, all your senses are needed to evaluate the terrain and handle the crutches or other mobility aid. Sobriety and stairs are particularly endorsed.

Casters and wheels: Be careful not to grab or use for support anything on casters or wheels: stools, tables, carts, or whatever.

Nighttime trekking: If fearless frolicking on urban or suburban by-ways is on your schedule, increase the likelihood that others will see you by sticking strips of luminous tape to your crutches or other mobility aid. A jogger's reflective vest is also highly recommended.

Hints for Independence

Portable phone or phone with an answering machine: If you expect to be laid up for a fairly long time, see if you can get one of these conveniences. It is a luxury that is worth its purchase price many times over, saving much getting up and down, and therefore *lots* of precious energy.

You will also be spared the frustration of having the phone hung up during innumerable struggles to reach it in time. In warm weather, a portable phone will allow you more recuperative opportunities outdoors, a valuable bonus for your overall physical and psychological recovery. By the time you are back on your feet, the status of your portable phone will probably have changed from a luxury to a necessity.

If you have a fixed phone and no answering machine, alert expected callers to let the phone ring a long, l-o-n-g time.

A is for apron: For women and men equally, this cryptic heading contains just about the single most valuable tip you will get from this book in terms of the desired goals of self-sufficiency and independence—even of safety. The whys and the wherefores, along with the hows, are to be found on the first page of Chapter 13, which you are highly encouraged to look at before too many hours or days of struggle have passed by.

Use of your good leg as a tool: Besides totin' you so many places, your uninjured leg can become an innovative implement in ways that are limited only by your own situation and need for innovation. It can pull things toward you, kick things away, arrange a sheet or blanket over the hump of your swollen knee on its pillows, and — placed underneath the broken leg — can lever or lift it, cast and all, to a more comfortable position.

Responsibility of the mobility-impaired person: It is up to you to let other people know when you need help — and how to provide it.

Sense of humor: Find it, use it. Here's one philosopher's advice: measure your situation on the "ladder of suffering" that exists for everyone. No matter where you are on that ladder, there are those below who are better off and *always* others *above* who are worse off. Humor reasserts realism; it helps prevent you from thinking you are at the top of the ladder of suffering, and it dissuades you from comparing yourself only to those who are better off below. Forget feeling sorry for yourself and . . . laugh.

Doctors have recently decided laughing is good for you — not only will deep-seated belly shakes cause you no harm, they will actually release tension, establish positive moods, and speed recovery. Use your good humor to "measure" your situation; the results will reward not only you but your family and friends as well.

One area you can focus on is the "Department of Snappy Answers to the Never-Ending Question of 'What Happened to You?' " Recounting details of accident or surgery — or worse yet, accident *and* surgery — can get exceedingly repetitious and tedious, especially if months of recovery and rehabilitation are involved. It's up to you to come up with some "good ones." Surely you will enjoy replying that using crutches is a personal solution to the need of building upper-body strength. Or that you're a halfback for the San Francisco 49ers (substitute any local big-name football team) and got blindsided on a downfield run (especially effective coming from women of a delicate build). Think of your own way to blindside the question "what happened?"

Pain, control: Research done at Stanford University Medical School shows there are two components to pain: the sensation itself and how much attention a person pays to it. Keeping busy — focusing on other things and other people — is crucial in getting through this period.

Patient-doctor relationship: Ideally, you and your physician are partners, and savvy consumers interview doctors before selecting one. However, unless you are planning elective surgery, it is unlikely you had a chance to assess your orthopaedic guru for qualities important to you, whether it's compassion, up-front "feeding of facts," or whatever. If you have time, by all means get a second opinion and check out the compatibility quotient of different doctors at the same time.

Be totally up front yourself about whatever your needs are—for thorough explanations, for updating of information, for basic emotional support, or fears of any kind. Modern medicine with its enormous complexity has brought about a fragmentation of care among multiple specialties, so it is unlikely that you will be cared for by a doctor who has known you all your life.

Do not be cowed; those in the medical professions are not gods, nor are they the perfect paragons portrayed on TV. Like men and women in any other occupation, physicians have their quota of winners and not so winning. As much as possible, educate yourself—be as cautious a consumer as you would be with any other service you are buying—realizing that some of the responsibility for your welfare is yours. Such preparation, providing a sense of control, has been found to lessen tension and significantly speed recovery.

Elective surgery, getting in shape, getting familiar with crutches: Those in good physical condition recover from injury and surgery faster—and place less burden on those that care for them. Knowing of pending surgery should galvanize you into action: get as fit and as flexible as feasible. Likewise, get fitted and fit with your crutches now, before you need them. You will be congratulating yourself for your foresight in weeks to come.

Getting Your Lifestyle Organized

Although *Getting Back on Your Feet* will save you untold energy and all sorts of hassle and frazzle, you can do a lot for yourself by being alert and aware. Evaluate your methods of doing each task and develop personal routines that simplify and satisfy your individual and particular lifestyle. Some people will find this more difficult than others, but do be attentive to the possibilities of making life easier on yourself. Considering the many situations you *can't* control, smoothing your own way won't be all that easy, even when you try.

Think things out in advance: Take what you need with you the first time, so as not to have to laboriously return and get it; make phone calls ahead that will save unnecessary steps or impossible parking; have clothing chosen and laid out before the last minute. *Plan ahead.*

Become an efficiency expert: Streamline your chores, pinpoint unnecessary steps, and analyze the simplest and fewest actions it takes to accomplish a given task. If the old way of doing something tires you out — or hurts — find another way. There may be certain jobs that really don't have to be done, and if there are essential ones that you just can't manage on your own, offer to do something — today, next month, or later — for a neighbor or family member in return for his helping you out now.

Do it right, do it well: If you *are* going to make an effort of any kind, make it in such a way that your energy will not be wasted in having to do it again.

Establish priorities: You can't do everything when dealing with an immobilizing injury, and certainly not in the same amount of time as you used to require. Decide what's important and what's not important, what's possible and what's impossible — in your work, your home, your personal care, your exercise routines, and your recreation. Be realistic. Choose some, let others go.

Tips about Time

With your life so much more restricted than previously, friends, relatives, and acquaintances will wonder what you do with "all that time."

The most basic guideline of all is never to forget that everything you do will take you a lot longer than it used to, a *whole lot* longer — because little chores are now large challenges.

As the days pass, routines do become easier, and if you're clever, you become more organized — but, even at your most advanced stage of crutch or assistive-aid expertise, you will generally need to plan on doubling previous time allotments. Triple them to start with.

(*That's* what you'll be doing with "all that time.")

Using *Getting Back on Your Feet*

The chapters of *Getting Back on Your Feet* are self-contained so that you can instruct yourself on any problem that is hindering your adaptation to limited mobility without having to read the preceding chapters.

Exercise for Recovery: Getting Started on the Road Back

3

By the time you reach this chapter, you'll have already learned there's a lot more you can do while dealing with a bum leg than you originally thought, and that is certainly true for exercise as well. Most of us think that injury, surgery, a cast, or some other type of restrictive situation means just that—restriction from exercise and activity forever—or for interminable weeks of sitting around waiting for something to heal. It may sound pretty enticing, all that goofing off, but plow on a bit further to make sure that the goof-off is going to be as great for you as you think.

You'll find it's just the opposite. If you're now stuck to stumbling around with some type of assistive device—yet were accustomed to being active and don't want to lose muscle tone and flexibility, you'll have to work on it. And if you were sedentary before, you might want to change your ways. You, more than a former fitness freak, will need to build up your strength and endurance so that on your first long walk—with or without help of some kind—you don't poop out before you've reached your destination.

Start now. The sooner you start, the better, for muscles begin to lose strength and bones their calcium within 24 hours of total bed rest. (A little more than a week in bed, and your heart output declines 16 percent.) *Each day of immobility will take two days of exercise to regain lost function and strength.* Put another way—by Dr. James Garrick in his informative book, *Peak Condition*—deconditioning occurs at five times the rate it took you to get into condition. He goes on to say, "If you hurt yourself, find a healthy way of continuing to exercise . . . the longer you're out, the harder it is to get back." Suggestions follow, and they are limited only by what you can dream up for yourself, your own particular situation, and your doctor's restrictions.

Note: Check with your doctor and physical therapist for approval of any exercise program.

● ● ●Word to the Wise: DOCTORS AND EXERCISE. A recent study found that less than 10 percent of doctors suggest to patients how they can exercise the *rest* of their bodies when one part is injured, despite the fact that disuse shortens and stiffens muscle fibers all over. "Secondary pain"—unrelated to the injury—occurs in unused healthy muscles and causes avoidance of exercise just when it is needed most, both for damaged and healthy areas. So you might have to point out to your doctor that you don't want *every* muscle to atrophy—just the ones that are out of commission because of injury.

On a related point, if you are scheduled to have elective surgery, a savvy way to help your recovery is to get in as good shape as possible beforehand. As Dr. James Rippe of the University of Massachusetts Exercise Laboratory states, "Without a doubt if you're in good physical condition you'll recover more quickly from illness or injury." (*Staying* in good shape is, therefore, an inexpensive form of medical insurance.) Familiarizing yourself with the exercises that you'll be doing postoperatively can also be advantageous.

Exercise and emotional recovery: Coming back physically from an accident and coming back mentally—particularly in career-threatening injuries—can be much the same thing. As essential as exercise is for muscle maintenance during immobilizing injury, it is almost more important for emotional and mental maintenance. Suddenly losing the ability to to get around freely or play a favorite sport can be a monumental blow. Writes Dr. Robert Brown of the University of Virginia Medical School, "Nobody knows exactly why exercise has an anti-depressant effect, but in part it's the psychological phenomenon of being able to set realistic goals and achieve them." Although your favorite sport may be out for now, the exercises that follow give you plenty of realistic and achievable goals. So get busy—whatever you do will help these weeks and months pass with less frustration and stress—and generate the positive moods and optimism needed at this time.

GUIDELINES FOR EXERCISING

Scheduling: Regaining physical strength, flexibility, and endurance takes time—a lot of it. Expect to make recovery a full-time job for quite awhile. Schedule exercise sessions just as you would other daily activities such as meals. Check with your doctor and once cleared for exercise, get geared up, get working. If possible, get geared up and working several times a day—multiple exercise sessions are better for keeping circulation pumping vigorously as well as muscles and joints limber.

Breathing: Do not hold your breath when doing your exercises. Working muscles need fuel, which comes from burning fatty acids and glucose in the presence of the oxygen provided by breathing. Breathing irregularly forces muscles to use another method to get energy, one that produces lactic acid, a waste product that hastens fatigue. So—inhale during recovery, exhale during the action—the best way to oxygenate working muscles.

Warming up: Choosing appropriate exercises from below, warm up slowly—not at full exertion—to achieve a body temperature at which muscles will be more elastic and less susceptible to injury.

Performing exercises: How you perform each exercise is more important than how many you do. Doing an exercise improperly both wastes time and risks further injury.

Stretching: Flexibility exercises are done *after* muscles are warmed up—slowly, without bobbing, and conservatively. They are *not* a personal test of how far you can go. The macho saying "No pain, no gain" is now a "no-no": no longer macho, it's considered stupid and prehistoric. Don't overdo; flexibility takes time to achieve, especially if you have mainly focused on a single sport for many years.

Performing stretches: Technique is very important. Ideally, stretching should take you to a point of tension that is very gentle, one that you feel but that does not hurt. This is held for 10–30 seconds. Next you move a fraction of an inch farther in the direction of the stretch until a mild increase in tension is felt. This is the developmental part of the stretch, also held for 10–30 seconds.

At either stage back off if tension or discomfort intensifies, because overstretching actually causes contraction of the very muscles you are trying to lengthen. Stay relaxed: breathe deeply and rhythmically while keeping the jaws slightly ajar. Repetitions are from two to five times.

Pacing: Start slow, always. There is a Zen concept, expressed as "learning to wait properly," that suggests focusing on long-term goals rather than on short-term ones. Applied to recovery, the principle is *patience:* don't rush to do something for which your body is not prepared. The number-one problem exercisers of all experience levels have is overdoing—either when just beginning, when resuming after a layoff, when starting a new sport, or when doing a new calisthenic exercise. Always start slow, stay conservative, be it with repetitions or weight, and add on to either in small increments. Professionals recommend starting out with 10 repetitions of a particular exercise—and working up to three sets of 10, but if 10 reps is too many to start with, do fewer. Muscle stiffness will be none or minimal this way, you won't work yourself to exhaustion, and above all, you're more likely to stick with your exercise program.

Caution: Remember that a recovering body not only requires a proper selection of exercise but also a slower pace in that exercise than a healthy one. Warning signals of pain or excessive fatigue should be signs to ease up—but not to stop exercising entirely. If, for some reason, you must quit your exercise program—now or at any time in the future—always, to avoid reinjury or new injury, resume at a lower level of intensity than the level you had reached when you stopped.

Cooling down: Do not stop an aerobic activity suddenly. Muscles are pumping stations for a substantial portion of the blood required by the heart. A hasty turn-off means they are no longer providing adequate contractions for distribution, so that blood pools in the vessels below the waist and blood supply for the heart is drastically reduced. Cool down gradually instead—five minutes of walking after running, treading water or walking in the shallow end of a pool after lap swimming, or relaxed cycling.

Varying your exercises: Variety helps in maintaining motivation. Extra exercises have been included so that you can choose some for your morning workout and do the rest for your afternoon workout. Reverse the order the next day. Be innovative. Put on motivating music. Do *not* put on television. TV is distracting, definitely inhibits maximum workout, and prevents proper execution of precise exercise.

● ● ●Word to the Wise: VIDEOTAPES. There are a number of exercise videotapes on the market that provide real help in the battle against boredom. They offer visual demonstration of many exercises similar to the ones here, along with the stimulation of hearing energetic music and watching energetic bodies—in fantastic shape—doing all the things you're trying to do. Some videos, although designed for sedentary senior citizens, are perfect for persons who are recovering from leg injuries or surgery, because the exercises are performed while holding on to a chair or walker. You can work up a pretty good head of steam even if you do have to hold on to something, which people with ankle, knee, hip, or foot injuries usually have to do. See Chapter 19 for details on videotapes.

BED EXERCISES FOR ARMS AND SHOULDERS

A lot of space has been devoted to these exercises because if your injury requires use of crutches, your arms and shoulder musculature will have to lift and then swing your entire body weight forward with each step. Your attention to conditioning now, when you're still confined to bed in the hospital or at home, is going to pay off in the near future. All these exercises can, of course, be continued throughout your recovery.

Biceps lifts: If the bed is equipped with an overhead orthopaedic frame — in a hospital it probably is — you can use the apparatus to work the important biceps muscles in the front of your arms. Raise yourself slowly up, and lower yourself slowly down, either using the arms together or one at a time. Start off with low repetitions and increase as your endurance permits.

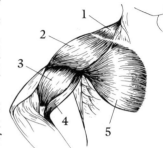

1 Trapezius
2 Deltoid
3 Biceps brachii
4 Triceps brachii
5 Pectoralis major

• • •Word to the Wise: ORTHOPAEDIC FRAME. If your injury makes it especially difficult to get out of bed, and you expect to be in that situation for an extended length of time, a portable overhead trapeze frame can be obtained from your medical-supply store. It can either be a floor model or be attached to the headboard.

Forward and reverse circles, extensions, "crawl stroke": The triceps muscles of the arms and depressor muscles of the shoulder are important in using crutches. Circles and extensions are part of everyday actions but are included here to give you exercises for good upper-body warmup as well as the stimulus and fun of easy and nondemanding movement for immediately after injury or surgery. *Circles.* In a sitting position, with the arms straightened to either side, do large circles, reaching forward and as high, low, and wide as your position permits. *Extensions.* Extend the arms directly in front, bring them slowly straight out to the sides, and return slowly. Alternate by extending to the sides, raising up toward the ceiling, and lowering. *Crawl stroke.* In a sitting position, Indian-style if feasible, do the overhand — "crawl" — swimming stroke, an active extension. Done moderately, this will give a pleasantly energetic feeling. You'll start feeling better even with simple exercises like these — as well as being warmed up for what's to come.

Triceps lifts: This is strongly recommended for the triceps muscles at the back of the arms, essential for using crutches. Raise one arm straight up and then bend the elbow over the head, with the hand pointing to the opposite shoulder. Hold a few seconds, lower and raise the other arm. Repeat.

To increase the workout, cuff weights can be put on each wrist, starting at one pound and working up. An alternative method is to take a cane in both hands, raise the cane over your head, followed by lowering it; add cuff weights to the cane if desired. A cane with or without weights can be used for other exercises as well and lends needed variety. Be innovative.

Shoulder shrugs: In a sitting position, hands at sides, raise your shoulders upward toward your ears. Lower, relax, and repeat. Holding a weight in each hand or using cuff weights is a good addition to this exercise.

Hand interlace: If you're lying around a lot, this stretch will make your whole upper body feel better—shoulders, arms and back. Sitting up (or later on, standing), lace your fingers above your head, palms up. Pushing your arms slightly back and up you'll get a pleasant lengthening of tight muscles. Another sitting stretch: interlace your hands, palms up, behind your back while lifting them back and up. A variation is to slowly turn your elbows inward while straightening the arms.

Windmill: Lying down with your good knee bent and the foot flat on the bed, put one arm above your head palm up and the other along your side palm down. Reach in opposite directions at the same time in a controlled motion. The stretch should be held 8–10 seconds. If speeded up from time to time you can create some light enjoyable exercise for your upper body.

Elbow scoot: Lie on your back and prop yourself on your elbows. Scoot your trunk and legs forward to get the stretch, which you will feel in front. Do not do the elbow scoot if you have had any shoulder injuries.

Prone push-ups: Lying on your stomach, place your palms close to your shoulders with the fingers pointing to the head of the bed. Push down on your hands, and straighten your elbows to lift the head and trunk. The body should be kept straight, with the hips and knees extended and in contact with the bed. If appropriate to your situation, you can bend the knees. This is an awkward exercise for most leg conditions but is included for those who are able and willing.

Weight lifts for triceps and biceps: Lying on your back, or sitting when you feel up to it, take a book or a can of soup in each hand and raise them directly up toward the ceiling to exercise the triceps. Raise slowly until your arms are almost straight, then lower even more slowly until your elbows are back resting on the bed. For the biceps, sit up with your elbows at your sides, hands with weights directly out in front of your body. Lift or curl the weights inward toward your shoulders. The size of the cans can be gradually increased (Campbell's soups are about 11 ounces), but if lifting any new amount of weight is too strenuous, back off or just raise part way.

● ● ●Word to the Wise: BARBELLS. If you are going to be slowed down for quite awhile, you can borrow or buy barbells. Should you be using crutches, arm and shoulder strength will be essential in the coming weeks; even when crutches are not your lot, you may not want to let your upper-body strength deteriorate. Barbells will help; they are available in one-pound weights and on up, suitable for both men and women.

As soon as you are able to perch on the side of the bed, the seven exercises just described will be more effective plus easier to do. Many of them can be done in addition to exercises performed at physical therapy or done at other stages of your recovery.

Seated push-ups: Once you're out of bed, this is the most important exercise of all, because it is the only one that works on both the triceps and the shoulder depressors — crucial if you'll be using crutches. And isn't it fortunate to have an exercise that works two essential muscle groups at the same time?

Whatever chair is used, it must have arms and be sturdy. Place your hands on the armrests, then push down on them until the arms are fully extended. Be sure to depress the shoulders — do *not* hunch them up — and tuck your buttocks in underneath the pelvis. Depending upon shoulder and abdominal strength, the legs may be raised horizontal to the floor or rest on the edge of the chair. Bend your elbows slowly to lower your body, relax, repeat.

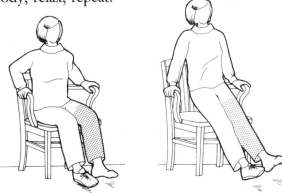

**Exercise
for Recovery:
LEGS**

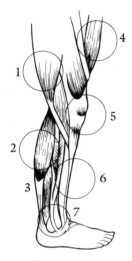

1 hamstring area
2 calf muscle area
3 Achilles tendon
4 quadriceps
5 knee area
6 shin area
7 ankle

Exercises for the injured leg must, of course, be ordered by your doctor, and usually are, even when the leg is in a cast or brace. If that's the good news, the bad news is that you have to strengthen the other leg also. Its future holds a lot of extra, unaccustomed work.

Exercises for the extremities must aim for proper muscle balance. Athletes frequently don't realize that there are two sets of muscles used in any one action: those that perform it, and those that provide stabilization and opposition or resistance. Injuries often occur because in concentrating on a single sport one muscle group (generally the performing one) is exercised to the exclusion of the opposite muscle group. The performing muscle group — disproportionately stronger than its counterpart — tends to shorten and tighten, making it prone to injury. The only way to remedy this situation is to strengthen the weaker muscle group and *stretch* the stronger one. Better yet is to keep unequal muscle development from happening in the first place by muscle balancing: the glamor-grabbing quadriceps at the front of the thigh are opposed by the hamstrings at the rear, adductors go up against the abductors (the inner and outer muscles of the thigh), shin muscles on the front of the lower leg counteract calf muscles behind, and ankles have their opposites on either side. Always, always pay equal attention to both.

Note: Crosstraining — employing varied training methods as well as playing other sports besides your dominant one — also counteracts muscle imbalance.

Caution: Depending upon your own particular situation, some of these exercises may not be appropriate or possible for you at this time. Check with your doctor or therapist for approval. In most cases, only the uninjured leg will be exercised to start with, and the injured leg added as your recovery progresses.

For ease in remembering, these leg exercises start with the muscle groups closest to your trunk and progress outward: buttocks, hips, upper leg, knee, lower leg, ankle, and foot.

Buttocks Strengthening

Buttocks squeezes: Lie on your back or supported on your elbows, with legs straight. Squeeze your buttocks together as tightly as possible. Hold, relax, repeat.

Prone knee lifts: Lying on your stomach, bend your knee to 90 degrees, lift it off the supporting surface three to five inches, hold, lower slowly, and repeat.

Buttocks raises: If both knees can bend, lie on your back and place your feet flat on the bed. Tighten your abdominal muscles, then curl the pelvis inward, and raise the buttocks. Hold, lower slowly, repeat.

Hip and Thigh Strengthening

Side leg raises for hip abductor muscles: "Abduct" means to take away—as in abducting someone. Thus the abductors move your leg *away from* the midline of the body. Lie on your side and slowly raise your upper leg straight up, keeping your hip and knee straight. Raise it about one foot, but not so far as to make a right angle with the bed. Lower slowly, relax, and repeat. Do the other leg if possible. The abductor/adductor muscle groups can frequently be out of balance when the dominant sport is aerobics, dance, or ice skating.

Towel squeezes for hip adductor muscles: The adductors are on the inside of the thigh and oppose the abductors. Sit on a firm surface with your hands behind you for support. Place a rolled towel between your legs. Keeping them straight, squeeze the towel between both legs. Hold a few seconds, relax, and repeat.

Side leg raises for hip adductor muscles: Lying on your side, cross the upper leg over the lower leg by bending the knee and placing the foot flat on the bed next to the lower knee. Keeping your lower leg straight, lift it slowly up toward the knee above. Lower. Repeat.

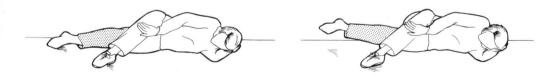

Hip leg raises for hip extensor muscles: Lying on your stomach, raise each leg alternately above the level of your buttocks. Keep the leg straight and your hands at your sides.

Hamstring Strengthening

Sports which involve running tend to overdevelop the quadriceps on the front of the thighs, so if that's your game don't neglect the counterbalancing hamstrings at the back.

Bent leg raises: Lie on your stomach, with hands folded under your face for comfort. While bending your knee, slowly bring the heel toward your buttocks. Lower it very slowly and hold briefly at the bottom of the action before raising again. If you are recovering from a knee injury, get clearance for doing this exercise. Later on, wearing a hiking boot or a weight makes these raises more productive; when you do this, you'll find the exercise is easier to do by starting with the weighted foot dangling slightly over the end of the bed.

Hamstring presses: Lie on your back, either flat or supporting yourself on your elbows. Alternately press the heel of each leg into the mattress, hold, relax, repeat. Or bend your good knee to a height of approximately six inches, heel into mattress, toes pointing up. Tighten the knee by digging down and back with the heel. Hold for a few seconds, relax, and repeat. If you have knee problems, get approval first.

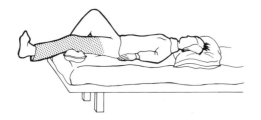 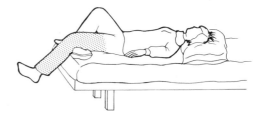

Knee Strengthening

Quadriceps sets: Isometric exercises — tightening of various muscle groups — can be done at any time and are particularly beneficial for the muscles in the front of the thigh. The quadriceps muscles keep the knees from buckling during the striding phase of walking. In learning to properly isolate the quadriceps muscle, place a small pillow or folded face towel under the knee, with the leg extended. Tighten the leg muscles by pressing the knee down into the pillow, and hold for a count of 10. The muscles above the knee will tighten and bulge. With practice you won't need the help of the pillow. "Quad sets" can be done anywhere, either lying down or sitting in a chair with the leg extended, and should be done as often as possible. They even can be done with the leg in a cast; take that opportunity to wiggle the toes as well.

Straight leg raises for the quadriceps muscles: Lying flat on your back, or reclining on your elbows, bend your good knee and place the foot flat on the bed. Straighten the injured leg as much as possible, tightening the muscles on top of the thigh. Raise it slowly 12–18 inches, toes pointed upward or slightly outward. Hold for several seconds, then lower slowly, relax, and repeat. Do the good knee, too, so it doesn't get lazy and flabby. (This is the workhorse rehabilitation exercise for the knee.)

Short-arc quads: Lie on your back with your legs straight. Place a tightly rolled pillow (or three-pound coffee can) under the knee of the leg to be exercised. Gradually straighten the knee by lifting the heel off the mattress, toes pointing up. Hold, lower slowly, relax, repeat.

Medium-arc quads (or bent leg raises):   Sit up or lie on your back, positioned so that your knees are at the edge of the bed, the foot of the leg to be exercised dangling over, the other leg bent with the foot flat near the edge of the bed. (If it's casted, the other leg will be straight—perhaps resting on a chair.) A rolled towel or pillow is placed under the leg to be exercised. The foot is dangling, not pointed directly at the floor—in order to restrict the distance of lift ("medium arc"). Slowly raise the foot to horizontal, hold, and lower. When appropriate add ankle weights.

Shin Muscle Strengthening

This area is badly neglected by the average fitness fanatic. Sitting with your feet on the floor, raise the toes, lower and tap the floor, repeat. (Later on, when you're walking again, assume a sprinter's starting position with your hands on the floor and one leg stretched back. Tap the toes of the front foot several times. Switch legs, repeat.)

Ankle and Foot Strengthening

Although the ankle is the most frequently injured joint, most people don't include it in their workouts. And while your present injury may not be an ankle one, if you are going to be non-weight-bearing you need to build up the ankle strength of your healthy leg. The moral is, of course, not to let the foot and ankle get off scot free. Flexing, extending, and rotating are their lot and should be started when you begin exercising for recovery.

Toe points and rotations: Lie on your back with knees straight. Bend your ankle(s), point your toes at your head, and hold for a few seconds. Point the toes in the opposite direction and hold. Relax and repeat. For rotation, turn your feet in circles, both clockwise and counterclockwise.

Theraband tugging: With your legs dangling over the side of the bed, place a heavy rubber band or a piece of surgical tubing around your feet. Keeping the heels together, pull the front of your feet apart. Reverse, keeping the toes together and pulling the heels apart. Repeat. Tubing and Theraband are available from medical-supply stores, or see Chapter 19 for mail-order options.

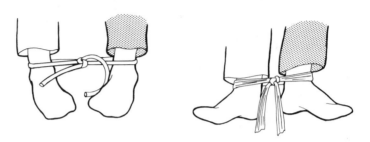

BED EXERCISES TO STRETCH THE LEGS

If permitted by your doctor, stretches are particularly important for the hamstrings and calf muscles.

Buttocks Stretches

Man-style: Sitting down, lift one leg and cross it man-style, placing the ankle on the opposite knee. Hold the ankle there and bend forward until you feel the stretch. Switch legs and repeat.

Hip and Thigh Stretches

Hip flex: Lie on your back and bring your knee(s) to your chest. Keep one knee pressed to the chest and stretch the opposite leg straight. Lower bent leg and repeat, alternating legs.

Hip extension: Lie on your stomach, hands under head, and raise your leg six inches off the mattress. Hold, lower, repeat and alternate.

Stretch for groin adductor muscles: Lie on your back with knees bent and feet together. Let each leg lower to the side so that they are flat on the mattress or gently press downward. The soles of the feet will be facing each other. Hold, relax, and repeat.

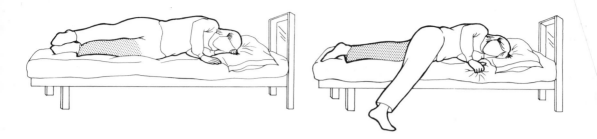

Stretch for outer thigh muscles: Lie on your side on the injured leg (if possible) near the edge of your bed. Keeping the top leg straight, raise it and move it forward and drop it off the side. Hold, raise, relax, and repeat. For better stability, hold on to the mattress. Do not do this stretch if your sense of balance is poor.

Hamstring Stretches

Seated hamstring stretch: Sit up straight with both legs extended. An injured knee may have a small pillow underneath. Tilt your lower abdomen/pelvis and lean gently forward, pressing the extended legs downward into the mattress until you feel a stretch. Do not force this position, do not attempt to touch your toes, and keep your back straight. Return to starting position, relax, repeat, and alternate with the other leg if possible. This stretch is also good for your lower back, counteracting some of the aches induced by bed rest.

Reclining hamstring stretch: Lie on your back with knee bent and the foot placed flat on the bed. (If the leg is casted, place a pillow under it.) Raise the other fully extended leg in the direction of your chest. Grasp and gently pull, keeping it *straight*. Return to start, relax, repeat, and alternate if possible. This exercise is for those with already good hamstring flex.

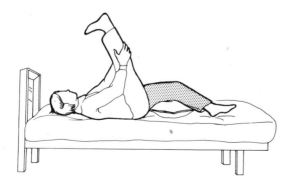

Knee Stretches

Quadriceps: Lie on your stomach, and bend one leg up toward your buttocks. With the hand on the opposite side of the bent leg, grab the ankle and gently pull it closer to the buttocks. Hold, lower, repeat.

> *Note:* Some knee conditions present such a limited range of motion that you will be unable to grasp your ankle. Looping a belt around the ankle and then pulling on it will keep those important quadriceps muscles from getting even tighter and risking other injury. Get your doctor's permission before doing either variation of this stretch.

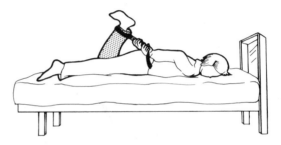

Calf Stretches

Calf muscles: Either sitting up or lying on your back, extend your leg(s) with the foot pointing up and make the toes point back in the direction of your knee. Hold for a couple of seconds, let them relax, then repeat.

BED EXERCISES FOR THE ABDOMEN

Strong stomach muscles are essential in prevention of back strain, which leg injuries and use of mobility devices can promote. Although not ideal, abdominal exercises can be performed in bed. (Unfortunately, constant compromising in all areas of recovery will become a fact of life—now and possibly for a long time.)

> *Caution:* When doing abdominal exercises, the back always should be kept flat and the pelvis and hips kept pressed to the mattress.

Abdominal Exercises

Pelvic tilt: The simplest of abdominal exercises, but very effective. With arms crossed on your chest, lie on your back, the good leg bent and foot flat on the mattress. (A pillow may always be placed under the injured leg.) Tighten your abdominal muscles while pushing your back down against the bed. Hold for several seconds, relax, and repeat.

Head raise ("toe stare"):   Another very easy one. Simply lie flat on your back—without your pillow and with arms at your sides. Keep your good knee bent, foot flat on the mattress, and do not arch your back. Slowly raise your head a couple of inches so that you are looking at your feet, while simultaneously tightening your abdominal muscles. Hold, lower, and repeat.

Advanced head raise: Bend your good knee and place the foot flat on the bed. With arms folded on your chest, slowly raise your head and look at your navel. Do not strain your neck forward. Hold for several seconds, then lower slowly. Relax. Repeat.

Stretching the Abdomen

Elbow raises: Lying on your stomach, place your forearms and hands just to the side of your body, and raise yourself on your elbows. Buttocks should be relaxed and floppy, hips should stay in contact with the mattress. Hold for a few seconds, lower yourself down, then repeat.

BED EXERCISES FOR THE BACK

Doing time in bed can make the back feel stiff and sore and downright painful. Stretches help relieve this discomfort as well as keeping you flexible and frisky for future frolic. There's variety here; pick and choose as you will.

Caution: If you have back problems of any kind, check with your doctor first.

Back Exercises

Lower back—trunk raises: Lying on your stomach, with arms alongside the body, raise your head and trunk from the mattress. Hold, lower, and repeat. For added effort place your hands behind your back, clasp them at buttocks level, and then raise. Harder still is placing your clasped hands behind your neck, but a firm surface is required.

Stretching the Back

Lower back – knee clasps: Besides stretching the back, this exercise also stretches hip flexors and knee muscles. Lie on your back and slowly bring your knee(s) to your chest. Clasp them with both arms, and pull gently back, holding for a few seconds. Lower, keeping the back flat, and repeat.

Lower back – trunk lean: Sit up straight, with a pillow under both knees. Tilting the lower abdomen, lean forward gently, chest up and arms outstretched horizontally. Do not force, do not touch your toes, keep your back straight. Return and repeat.

Trunk stretch: Sitting up, legs preferably dangling over the side of the bed, place your hands behind your head and rotate from the waist. Twist gently and thoroughly. This will make a bed-bound back feel great. When your situation permits, it can be done sitting in a chair or standing up.

Exercise for Fitness: Getting Strong, Flexible, Active — and Staying That Way

4

"If you don't exercise you pay the price . . . not just true for strength and endurance . . . [but also for] range of motion, cardiovascular health, your muscles' ability to contract and just about everything else you can think of," — so states Dr. James Garrick, author of *Peak Condition*. If you've had surgery, an uncomfortable fracture, or most any injury, you'll be made to get out of bed — probably — long before you, yourself, are feeling willing or able. It's a big step in the right direction, though — and a necessary one — to perk up your circulation and prevent dangerous blood clots. From now on your attitude, persistence, and the hours spent on exercise will determine how much freedom from dependence on others you can achieve. Physical stamina is an important part of this, so don't "hang out," get with it.

Review the beginning of Chapter 3 for guidelines on proper warmup and cool-down, breathing, stretching, repetitions, creating variety, and how best to incorporate any new exercise.

EXERCISES FOR THE INJURED AND UNINJURED LEG

If you've had a cast removed you have a vivid demonstration of what lack of exercise does to muscle and tissue. In six weeks or so a leg will appear 40 years older: weak, wasted, and wrinkled — demonstrating the effects of slowed circulation, loss of bone mass, and decreased range of motion. Luckily, you can and will be doing something about this.

Once mobile, willing or not, get up and use your crutches, cane, or other aid as frequently as your condition will allow, attempting to increase the distance you go each time, be it only a yard or so. The exercises included in this chapter are often stand-up versions of the ones in the previous chapter. Some of those routines are important to continue, others can be eliminated or kept, as you prefer — and done on the floor if you can comfortably get yourself there. Choose your favorites from each chapter, and with the variety provided you should be able to stay motivated.

With your doctor's or therapist's approval, most of the following exercises can also be done with ankle weights added. Depending upon your individual situation, the exercises are appropriate for both injured and uninjured limbs.

Hip and Thigh Strengthening

Standing hip extension for gluteal muscles: With good posture, stand facing a bureau or counter ledge that offers support, holding on with both hands. Keeping your body straight and upright throughout the exercise, move your injured leg back as far as possible. Keep the knee straight. Slowly return to start. Repeat.

Standing hip extension for abductors: With good posture, stand next to a bureau or counter ledge, holding on with one hand for support. Move the injured leg straight out to the side as far as possible. Keep the knee straight. Return, repeat.

Hamstring Strengthening

Standing hamstring curls: With good posture, stand facing a bureau or counter ledge. Support yourself with both hands. Bending your knee, slowly bring your heel to the buttocks. Lower slowly, relax, repeat. Weights can be added.

Quadriceps Strengthening

It takes strong leg muscles to have strong knees. Strong leg muscles and strong knees equal less chance of injury in the future—but only if you make sure the future includes working those muscles and knees. Most times, this means every day. Mostly, the best hour is the one when you get up (no matter how early). No excuses accepted for lack of time—simply get up 15 minutes earlier—nor for being too tired—you've just gotten up. It is a method that is almost failure-proof, so since neglect hurts no one but you, get motivated and get up.

Armchair stands: A simple but very good exercise to start with, especially if you're weak or have a cumbersome leg cast. A few stands can be slipped in any time you're sitting—an intriguing contradiction in terms. Using a firm armchair, slowly stand up, then slowly sit down, using the arm rests for help in the beginning.

Straight leg raises: Although described in the previous chapter, this exercise is so essential for the quadriceps that it is repeated here to be sure it's not overlooked. Lying flat on your back, or reclining on your elbows, bend your good knee and place the foot flat on the bed. Straighten the injured leg as much as possible, tightening the muscles on top of the thigh. Raise it slowly 12–18 inches, toes pointed upward or slightly outward. Hold for several seconds, lower slowly, relax, and repeat.

Sitting leg raises: Sit on a surface that is high enough so your feet don't touch the floor. Grip the front edge of the surface (whether countertop or chair seat) to prevent yourself from rocking or using your back and shoulders to help out. Straighten your knee completely, bringing it slowly from the dangling position—toes pointing up—to the horizontal position. Lower slowly, relax, repeat.

> *Caution:* Check with your doctor before adding weights, and do so cautiously, since excessive weight and repetitions can aggravate or cause knee-joint problems.

Ankle Strengthening

Rebuilding of ankle strength is often neglected in lower-extremity rehabilitation, which—considering the importance of the ankle—makes little sense. Strengthening is needed to prevent injury as well as to rehabilitate ankles after injury.

Heel raises: With good posture and feet shoulder width apart, hold onto a bureau or counter ledge for support. Push up on your toes, raising your heels as high as possible. Hold, lower slowly, and repeat. This exercise can also be done on one foot at a time. Progress to doing these raises on the edge of a book or a stair—with a banister for stability—either with one or both feet and with your heels being lowered below the level of the stair tread.

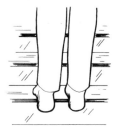

Toe raises, heel walk: Holding on to a support, raise your toes off the floor, one foot at a time or both feet at a time. Or, on your *heels* only, toes in air, "stagger" across your bedroom, kitchen, or wherever —gradually increasing the distance. You won't feel like the world's most coordinated athlete doing these, but maybe having done them, you'll be in a position to become one. Do these at least twice a day, especially after ankle injury.

Rotations: Sitting on a firm surface without your feet touching the floor, rotate your ankles in circles, going in both directions. Progress to using cuff weights.

STRETCHING THE INJURED AND UNINJURED LEG

If your injury has required casting or immobilization of any kind, stretches help prevent permanent contraction of affected joints. This is particularly important for knees—in which contraction shortens the leg—resulting in gait abnormalities, decreased speed of walking, and lessened shock absorption. Here are some additional stretches to those already described in Chapter 3. Incorporate plenty of variety to make it easier to stay with your program.

Hip Stretching

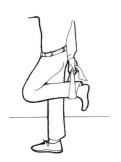

Standing stretch for flexors: Facing a bureau, ledge, or wall, support yourself with one hand. Bend back the leg on the same side as the hand you are supporting yourself with. Grasp the ankle with the opposite hand. Hold, lower, relax, repeat. This takes a certain amount of agility, and if you have knee or balance problems, should only be done with your doctor's approval. Looping a towel or belt around the ankle and grasping it instead of the leg itself makes this exercise easier to perform.

Hamstring Stretching

Sitting "astride" stretch: Sit on the floor with your back against a wall and legs out in front. Move your legs gradually outward to the sides. Keeping the back straight, lean a few inches forward, hold, relax, repeat.

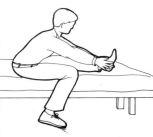

Sitting single-leg stretch: This is considered the best stretch for hamstrings but can be uncomfortable to start with. Don't give up; it will gradually get easier. Sit on the side of a bench, bed, couch, or counter with one leg straight on the surface and the opposite leg draped off the side. Keeping your back straight, lean forward and grasp the calf or ankle of the straight leg, pressing the leg into the surface at the same time. Hold, relax, repeat. Change position so that the opposite leg can be stretched. Repeat.

Lying-down stretch: This version of a hamstring stretch offers variety by virtue of the unique positioning: you can even read in comfort while doing it. In front of the doorway of your choice, lie on the floor with one leg through the doorway. Keeping the other leg straight, place it on the door frame. Scooch forward so that your buttocks, leg, and heel—toes pointing backward—are tight against the frame. Press the leg in, hold, relax, repeat. Enjoy your book.

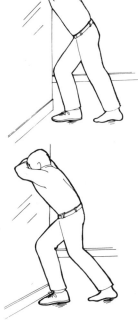

Calf Stretching

Tight (shortened) Achilles tendons (also called heel cords) lead to rupture, an injury that strikes the active athlete in particular. The Achilles tendon consists of two parts, the *gastrocnemius* (upper) and *soleus* (lower) muscles. The following exercises prevent tightening of both muscle groups and should be done for . . . forever.

Upper Achilles tendon stretch: Facing a wall, place your folded arms against it to support the upper trunk. Your feet should be about four to six inches from the wall. Move one leg back; press it backward and keep the knee straight. The foot should be flat, pointed forward, and slightly turned in. Let the other leg relax and bend the knee in naturally to touch the wall, with the foot kept flat. Hold, relax, repeat, and then alternate legs. You should feel pulling in the backs of your calves.

Lower Achilles tendon stretch: Facing a wall, bureau, or counter ledge, support yourself as in the above exercise or by holding on to the ledge. Your feet will be four to six inches from the wall. Move one leg back and instead of keeping the knee straight, bend it, and press forward. Be sure the foot is kept flat and pointed forward. Let the other knee relax and bend in the direction of the wall, foot kept flat. Hold, relax, repeat, and alternate legs. The stretch should be felt at the bottom of the calves.

ARM AND SHOULDER EXERCISES

It's helpful to realize that if your recovery requires use of crutches, your arms and shoulders will be providing two-thirds of your ambulatory *oomph* . . . so power them up now. These exercises are supplements to those you started with in Chapter 3, some of which should be done now as part of your upper-body warmup.

Free Weights

Light barbells are the best choice for these exercises, but cans of food in appropriate weights can also be used.

Triceps press: Hands at shoulder height, slowly lift weights straight up until your arms are fully extended. Lower slowly, repeat.

Biceps lift: Hands at waist level, elbows bent, slowly bring the weights to your chest. Lower slowly, and repeat.

Shoulder raise: Starting with your hands at your sides, slowly raise them until they are at shoulder height, elbows straight. Lower slowly, and repeat.

ABDOMINAL EXERCISES

The same exercises that were outlined in Chapter 3 for persons confined to bed can, of course, be done on the floor, and much more successfully. If your leg is casted or remains contracted in a flexed position, place a pillow under the knee for support. Then get on with the following exercises, some or all. Keeping abdominal muscles strong is crucial in preventing back problems.

Caution:

Never have both knees straight when doing abdominal exercises. Experts advise that keeping the knees flexed and feet on the floor avoids strain on the back, and better isolates the abdominal muscles.

Never clasp your hands behind your head when doing head raises combined with abdominal exercises. Such support tends to put dangerous presssure on bones, discs, and nerves in the neck.

Never place your feet under a bed or have someone hold your ankles, because the abdominals will not be isolated if you are restrained that way.

Abdominal curl: Lie on your back with your knees bent and feet flat. Using your hands to help pull yourself up, grab your thighs and raise your head two to three inches or until your shoulders are clear of the floor. Holding your legs increases your repetitions and eases the strain on neck muscles. When stronger, your hands can be kept at your side. For persons of intermediate fitness, arms can be folded on the chest. Rise only to the point where the lower portion of the shoulder blades clears the floor, and do not help yourself by holding on to your knees. Keep the lower back pressed flat. A small pillow under the neck is recommended for all abdominal curls.

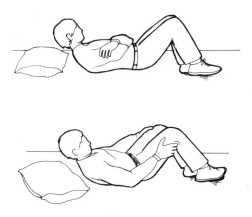

Spinal curl for lower abdominals: Lying on your back, place your hands under your buttocks, and bring your knees to your chest, keeping your stomach tight and back flat. Your lower legs — from knees to toes — should progress to a position parallel to the floor before lowering. Keep everything especially tight — and back pressed into the floor — as you lower the legs. Repeat.

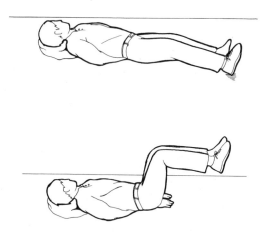

Chair crunch: Lying on your back, place both legs on a chair or bed, knees bent at the edge. (If necessary you can stick the injured leg under the chair or bed and put the good one up on it, knee bent at the edge.) Place your hands on your chest, and raise your head in the direction of your knees. (Holding on to your legs, behind the knees, will make this less demanding.) Hold, lower slowly, relax, repeat. A few repetitions, and the "abs" should let you know you are making an impact.

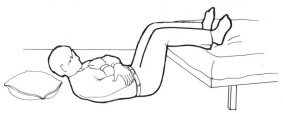

BACK EXERCISES

Chest raise, back extension: Lie flat on your stomach with your arms stretched straight ahead. Keeping your chin tucked in, raise your head and arms about one inch off the floor as you "pinch" your shoulder blades together. To prevent arching of the back, press pelvis and hips into the floor while raising. Hold, lower, relax, and repeat. This can also be done with your arms at your sides and a small pillow under your stomach to relieve back strain.

Stretch for lower back muscles: Lie on your back and bring your knee(s) to your chest. Clasping your arms around them, gently pull them in close. Hold, relax, repeat.

Remember, these and other exercises are only suggestions and additions to those in Chapter 3. Ideally, methods, guidelines, and above all precautions described here have inspired you to exercise conscientiously and safely. Desire plus determination plus execution will find you getting a pretty good workout after all.

EXTRA-CURRICULAR EXERCISE

Dependent upon your individual situation, after the initial recovery period you may have little spare time for anything but your job and/or taking care of your family and home. On the other hand, you may have plenty, so be on the lookout for athletic diversions besides the ones suggested here. In *Love, Medicine and Miracles*, Dr. Bernie Siegel encourages varied activity as pyschic therapy, writing that "all forms of exercise help you 'hear' your body and its needs while shutting out other concerns." Repetitive types of physical motion, like cycling, walking, or swimming—when you don't have to think about what you're doing—encourage reflection and mental exercise as well. Variety in exercise is essential to keep psyched up, revved up, and ready to try whatever comes your way.

Types of Exercise

There are several types of exercise, most of which you will probably be doing during your recovery.

Isometric exercise: You can do isometrics when you're just sitting or lying around since these exercises involve only alternate tightening and relaxing of muscles. With or without a cast, isometrics are invaluable for early rehabilitation and have great value as do-anywhere (office, train, plane, or couch) exercises. Quadriceps sets are an example.

Aerobic exercise: An aerobic exercise is one that uses large muscle groups continuously and for long enough to create a sustained oxygen demand that requires an increase of blood flow and oxygen throughout the body. It is activity that forces oxygen through the system and achieves training effects that include a stronger, more efficient heart, improved circulation, and better lung function. Aerobic activity is also thought to enhance brain function. Since the brain needs more oxygen than any other organ—20 percent of the available supply—exercise that increases oxygen supply is important for that reason alone. Running, swimming, brisk walking, and cycling for a minimum of 30 minutes are outdoor options. Treadmills, rowing machines, Nordic-Track, exercycles, and Stair Masters are indoor choices.

"Interval training" is a refinement of aerobic exercise technique. Rather than exercising at one sustained rate, sprints of the exercise being performed are alternated with a base rate. The sprints can last from 15 to 60 seconds depending on the activity and fitness level. Interval training is now believed to result in higher levels of cardiovascular fitness and can be employed in any repetititve form of endeavor from swimming to exercise machines.

Anaerobic exercise: Exercise of this sort does not increase blood flow significantly, either because the length of time the activity is done is too limited or because the muscle demand is of an isolated sort. Considerable as the heart rate may be, and considerable as the static muscular work may be, the exercise will be *an*-aerobic, *without* the forced oxygen dispersal that *sustained* exercise creates. Examples are weightlifting, horseback riding, sprints, and tennis, all of which are good sports and good for you, but are not aerobic.

● ● ●Word to the Wise: RELAPSES. Healing of knee, leg, and ankle injuries takes a long time. Naturally when you get back to walking and other former activities, you assume that your lengthy rest, recuperation, and rehabilitation have put your injured leg in top working order. Alas, despite your faithful rahabbing, newly resumed activities can put unaccustomed stress on the injured area, causing a bewildering variety of painful complaints for a good while to come. Be assured that each interim pain does not mean the operation wasn't a success or that the injury will leave you in permanent agony. Give each new activity multiple short tryouts, always expecting some initial discomfort. Such symptoms will probably subside as time passes — time is still "the great healer." At the end of a year look back, and you will probably recall a lot of alarming pains that just are not a factor anymore. At the end of two years, even the recall will be gone.

● ● ●Word to the Wise: POST-EXERCISE ICING. Icing of your leg in the affected area after exercise can reduce inflammation and pain due to the activity. Methods range from ice bags to joint-conforming wraps. See Chapter 2 for more about icing and do not neglect this aspect of long-term recovery.

Caution: When in doubt about any new pain or symptom, particularly one which persists, check with your doctor.

Crutching: Once you've gotten pretty stable on your "sticks," strength and stamina increase in proportion to how much you get out and around on them. So hit the sidewalks, the driveways, and the byways; go for walks or strolls, short at first, and keep lengthening the distance. Soon the body will be as ready as the spirit to go anywhere.

WORKOUT MACHINES AND FREE WEIGHTS

Machines rate a definite edge over free weights when you're rehabilitating a leg injury, since many free-weight exercises will have become impossible, too uncomfortable, or too risky. Machines allow you to train your entire upper body, the uninjured leg, and possibly both hips.

So — if you have access to a fitness facility — cast, crutches, or wheelchair should not keep you from using the machines, which are specifically designed to isolate and exercise individual body components. Setting seat heights and weights can be tricky at first, but those adjustments, and figuring out how to establish yourself on the various apparatuses, are just more hurdles that are not so impossible as they might seem.

Besides building up actual strength, most workout systems are designed to stretch muscle groups at the same time. As Dr. James Garrick emphasizes in *Peak Condition*, strength and range of motion coexist. "Regaining strength is as important in rehabilitating an injury as regaining range of motion—they go together." Fitness clubs are great in this respect, as well as being good places to find lots of different-size free weights for some of your own innovative, self-designed exercises.

● ● ●Word to the Wise: AGE. Don't let increasing years make you doubt the benefit of strength training after injury or surgery. Research shows that loss of strength and muscle mass are not inevitable and irreversible consequences of getting older. Biological age, the actual physiological condition of the body, can be dramatically improved by weight training whatever your *chronological* age—and this, of course, will help you bounce back quicker and more successfully to normal walking.

Although statistics vary, everyone starts—at age 25—to lose about a half pound of muscle per year. By age 45 this could figure out to as much as 5 to 10 pounds, and at age 60 as 20 percent of your original muscle mass!

You will probably not have lost weight, however, because fat cells replace the lost muscle. Muscle mass uses up more calories than fat: with less muscle to maintain, your metabolism slows down, and weight becomes increasingly difficult to control. Weight control is important in avoidance of muscular and skeletal injuries and reduction of stress on arthritic joints.

In addition, muscle mass is directly related to bone mass and density. A strength-training program will not only help muscle and bone recovery now but is equally important for long-term health of the entire body.

● ● ●Word to the Wise: GUIDANCE. Before starting training, get help from qualified instructors. Alert them to your situation and any medical restrictions. Be especially wary of repetitions or weight that *you* suspect may be excessive. Instructors are not infallible, are sometimes overly "gung-ho," and often have minimal training.

Above all, do not overdo. Fatigued muscles mean diminished strength and flexibility, promoting a risk that the activity (whether lifting weights, using an exercycle, or swimming laps) will require more of those goods than you have left. Do not risk aggravation of your present injury or a brand-new injury through ill-planned or excessive training.

Start with low weight amounts and few repetitions for *all* muscle groups — to avoid injury someplace else. Later on, when resuming your favorite sport, "bite the bullet" and restrict the amount of time you participate no matter what your eagerness and fitness quotient is — "them's *minutes* you start with," not hours. Like sunbathing, it's 15 minutes in the beginning — with *very* gradual increases on the road back to normal participation.

Exercycle

This machine gives you the opportunity for a real aerobic workout and is highly recommended for those anxious to maintain any semblance of cardiac and pulmonary fitness during recovery. It will also help in rebuilding endurance — which starts deteriorating within two days of injury.

As always, start slow, gradually increase the amount of time on the cycle, and then plan on 20–30 minutes a day to achieve any aerobic results. If you're ambitious "to get back fast," you might eventually want to do two daily sessions. To promote such effects be sure to use the toe clip — after your doctor or therapist has given permision. End with gentle stretching — good conditioning is useless if it is restricted by inflexible muscles.

Cycling with Casts or Braces

For leg injuries requiring casts or braces, exercycling need not be ruled out. Frank Shorter, a top American runner, taped his below-the-knee cast to the pedal and cranked away. Depending upon your situation you may be bicycling like Frank, or unicycling — using only one pedal. There are two methods to accomplish this, and your choice will probably depend on your injury and stage of recovery.

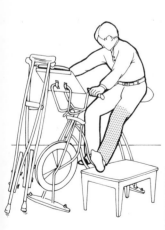

Injured leg not exercised: The casted leg is placed on a a high stool or chair to the side of the cycle, the tension regulator is set lower, and pedaling is done with the good leg. The seat height of the exercycle should be set so there is about a 15-degree bend in the working knee.

> *Caution:* Be careful to increase cycling time conservatively so as not to injure your healthy leg.

Injured leg exercised passively: The cycle seat is raised higher to accommodate the limb that should not be working or will not flex, be it due to limited range of motion, non-weight-bearing status, or whatever. The high seat prevents the injured leg from providing power or doing anything but rest on the pedal. Because, however, the seat height makes it hard to reach the working pedal, wear a thick-soled shoe on the foot of the good (power) leg or tape a small wooden block to the pedal. A foot stool may be necessary to help you climb aboard.

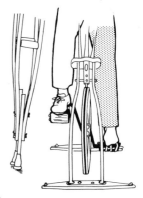

Since the injured leg most likely is just going along for the ride, to prevent it from inadvertently getting caught in the toe clip, tape the clip closed so the foot cannot enter. As only one leg provides pedaling power, wheel tension must be low. Exercycling will work out not only the heart and lungs but also—when the cast is removed—enhance circulation and range of motion of the injured leg. As range of motion improves, lower the seat accordingly to promote further flexibility.

Cycle entertainment: To up the amusement level of this type of cycling, now's the time to turn on the TV, invest in a book rack for your bike, or tune out with a Sony Walkman. For an alternative to music or TV, books on tape can be bought, borrowed from the library, or rented from video outlets.

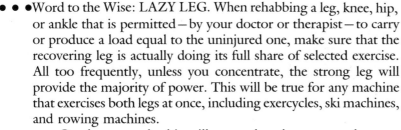

• • •Word to the Wise: LAZY LEG. When rehabbing a leg, knee, hip, or ankle that is permitted—by your doctor or therapist—to carry or produce a load equal to the uninjured one, make sure that the recovering leg is actually doing its full share of selected exercise. All too frequently, unless you concentrate, the strong leg will provide the majority of power. This will be true for any machine that exercises both legs at once, including exercycles, ski machines, and rowing machines.

On the exercycle this will mean that the stronger leg may downstroke so powerfully that it will provide most of the lift for the uprising weak leg. Ditto for the upstroke; the good leg will dominate the power ratio. *Concentrate on knowing and feeling how much power your weak leg is providing.* Another way to trick your recovering leg into more work is by removing the good foot from the pedal strap and letting *it* go along for the ride.

Note: Keep the cycle's wheel tension set low enough so that the weak leg *can* work up to its available capacity. Now, get inspired, get on board, and get going.

HAND/EYE COORDINATION:
KEEPING SPORTS SKILLS SHARP

No matter if playing a sport is a love or your livelihood—weeks in recovery wreak havoc not only with conditioning but with essential skills. The fields and courts are out of bounds for now, but practice of other kinds may be possible. A softball, football, beach ball, basketball, or medicine ball can be thrown overhand with one hand or overhead with both hands, pushed away, or pitched underhand—with the weight, types of throws, speed, and intervals of repetition being varied as desired. Sit wherever convenient: on a wall, a chair, a bed, the floor, or the ground.

Ping-pong can also be an option; a bar stool works well as a seat, a wheeled one would be ideal, or a wheelchair will work if one is available. (Some full-time wheelchair users are awesome at ping-pong.) Have lots of ping-pong balls on hand to keep the game lively—because *you'll* not be as lively at chasing the misses.

Mental-Imaging Techniques for Frustrated Athletes

A psychologist for the United States Olympic Committee says that mental practice of sports skills is highly effective in helping retain such skills—in fact, 40 to 50 percent as effective as real practice. ("If two groups of athletes stopped training in November, by March the group that mentally practiced all the time would have retained more skill.")

To make mental practice work for you, imagine yourself powerfully and totally involved in practicing the skills needed for your sport. Presto, neurons fire in the brain and trick your body into thinking it is doing something it isn't. After "practice," add the "real thing" with visualization of a competition, race, or match.

During your actual, repetitive, endurance-building, aerobic exercise, such as exercycle, swimming, or water walking, keep motivated by imagining more inspiring experiences—place yourself on a favorite road, course, ocean, lake, or whatever. Surprisingly, the imagined bliss need not be directly related to the drudgery you are actually doing.

WATER EXERCISE

Water-immersion activities are wonderful additions to your recovery: soft on joints, hard on muscles, and long on results. When the time is ripe, explore the accessibility in your area of Jacuzzis, hot tubs, and pools for swimming, aqua walking, and aqua running, and then, on the schedule your doctor or therapist has set for you, take advantage of them.

Many of the exercises previously described in this section can be performed more easily in water, because water support and body buoyancy make you weigh only 10 percent of true weight. Water exercise is extremely efficient, providing resistance in all directions — horizontally, vertically, and circularly — yet does not jolt or shock injured limbs. Water resistance also makes it harder to favor the recovering leg and promotes greater gains in range of motion. Make up your own exercise routines depending upon your particular situation.

> *Note:* Keeping your arms underwater, when possible, increases any workout effort.

Walking, running, and cycling in deep water, as alternatives to the various swimming strokes, are aerobic winners. A Wet Vest, Aqua Jogger, or life jacket that helps with buoyancy and maintaining an upright position is highly recommended. See Chapter 19 on where to obtain such aids.

Aqua walking: Water is an excellent place to practice and perfect normal gait patterns after an extended non-weight-bearing period or time in a cast. Once proper walking habits are restored, progress to energetic walking — moving arms and legs actively to build up strength and endurance. Aqua walking is done at the depth at which your foot can land normally.

Aqua running: If you are an injured runner, aqua running will get your pulse rate up and your body moving in a nice, familiar way again. Start with a slow, short jog, do your regular stretches, then return to a jog, concentrating on exaggerated arm and leg movements. Work up to interval sprints and longer endurance "runs." Running done in deep water is generally found more satisfying than shallow water, as the motion is closer to actual running.

Aqua cycling: In chest-deep water, simulate the pedaling motion of a bike — keep it up, and *that's* conditioning!

> *Caution:* Never take a steaming-hot shower, sauna, Jacuzzi, or hot tub after vigorous exercise. Blood vessels, already expanded from the workout, may dilate excessively. Wait at least five minutes after your workout and then use warm, not hot, water.

WALKING

When your recovery is almost complete, walking will most likely be incorporated into your return to fitness and fun. Unlike high-impact activities like running—in which your feet hit the ground with a force several times your body weight—walking is at a much kinder level of one and a half times body weight. Even if your love or livelihood is basketball or motorcycle racing, walking is quite literally a big step forward. Use an assistive aid in the beginning—follow the advice of your therapist—to retrain proper gait and to allow the recovering limb maximum participation. Gradually increase your pace and distance.

● ● ●Word to the Wise: WEIGHT. Weight impact and exercise are affected by body weight in general. Extra pounds *pound* and over-stress leg joints and structures with every step taken.

As with any repetitive exercise that is not done to excess, walking is a tool of relaxation. Long strides and good arm swings, the rhythmic action of placing one foot ahead of another, and the automaticity of it all create a nonstressful exercise that relaxes both mind and body. Walking is also supposed to beef up our immune system's defense cells, which helps our *overall* health—not bad for such a simple natural activity. Walking to music can increase both pleasure and pace for some participants.

● ● ●Word to the Wise: FOOTWEAR. When walking becomes a part of your therapy, buy shoes designated only for that—not for jogging, tennis, aerobics, or anything else. Such a shoe is specifically designed to reduce shock while walking—an obvious benefit for any limb or joint injury—increasing comfort and the ability to "put in distance." Having a sport-specific (walking) shoe is particularly important for women, whose heel strike—the angle and impact of the heel striking the ground—is proportionally greater than that of men.

After restricted mobility of any kind, it's very likely that your feet are no longer the tough creatures they used to be, with calluses in all the right places. Soft feet are ripe for blisters. Be alert for the chafing or burning sensations that indicate blisters—and immediately apply a band aid, or better yet, Moleskin or Molefoam. At least a half-inch of space between the end of your toes and the front of the shoe is also important.

STAIR CLIMBING

Climbing stairs has become a popular way of keeping fit, mainly through stair machines at health clubs. However, you can get some of the same advantages if you have stairs at home, and probably run a lot less risk of overdoing, something you should be wary of even at this advanced stage of recovery.

Step-ups: Find a small object such as a book or a board that will hold your weight. Step onto it with your injured leg, and fully straighten it. Step down, repeat. As leg strength improves, the height of the step can be raised. A single stair or level change can also be used for step-ups.

Stairs: When your condition permits, flights of stairs can be added to increase strength and endurance and to allow exercise during rainy or winter weather. Be careful not to overdo. Snappy music to step to is definitely a help here.

● ● ●Word to the Wise: PHYSICAL CONDITIONING. Good physical conditioning is a form of insurance against injury. To keep and build on what you have takes constant effort. Beware of the insidious traps and barriers, often mental, which follow. *Wintertime.* In addition to low temperatures, more hazardous outdoor conditions, and diminished choices, motivation is also negatively affected by the fewer hours of sunlight during winter. Since exercise has a positive psychological effect, physical activity is even more important to offset the gloom and dark of this season. *Lack of time.* Most people "don't have time" to exercise — until they have a heart attack. Then all of a sudden they do. Consider getting up earlier, utilizing lunchtime, parking farther away from your destination, whatever. 'Nuff said. *Too bored.* You've plain "had it": skipping your entire set of prescribed exercises has now become routine. Rather than complete avoidance, elect to do only one or two of the exercises each day, choosing a different one — or pair — the following day. One is better than none. *Too tired.* Determine only that your chosen exercise will go a very short distance or last a very short length of time — so short as to be laughable. See if at the limit you've set you're now set up for more, but don't do more. Add a little bit of time, a very little bit of distance — the next day. Willing to go just a very little way will get you going every day.

CROSSTRAINING

As you approach total recovery, a final reminder on the wisdom of alternating your athletic endeavors. Performing one sport exclusively builds up some muscle groups to the detriment of others, which leads to injuries ranging from strains to ruptures and possible future joint deterioration. Varying your fitness program prevents boredom from repetition and often enhances skills in the dominant or preferred sport.

5   Recovering with Crutches

Well, it's time to get started on the bread-and-butter bonanzas of life with mobility aids — how to subdue them, how to get around, how to work, and how to have fun. If it's crutches you're consigned to, you have probably already quickly surmised that they will not be high on your list of favorite possessions. This chapter and the following ones will render crutches and all aids a bit less antagonistic — I promise!

CRUTCH BASICS

In most cases, specific advice on technique in using crutches will be aimed at the non-weight-bearing person, that individual who is not allowed to place any weight on a leg, ankle, or foot. All other advice is applicable for mobility-impaired persons of all kinds, using aids of all kinds — as appropriate and indicated for individual disability, strength, coordination, age, judgment, or other limiting factors. When in doubt about any advice or technique, consult with your health professional. In all circumstances follow your doctor's orders.

Types of Crutches

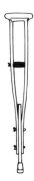

Crutches have been in use for five thousand years, and only recently has there been anything but underarm models. Your injury, physical condition, and age may dictate which type is prescribed. The most common of the models available are:

Axillary, underarm, or "double upright extension" crutches (wood model):   Most non-weight-bearing persons find the underarm type more stable and therefore less tiring than other designs. They can be bought at medical-supply stores or will be furnished by your doctor or hospital. The length and design of this type of crutch make it a useful tool in innumerable situations — to rest your injured leg on in various ways, for dragging and lifting objects (see Chapter 14), or for just hanging off of in tiring circumstances.

Underarm crutches also lend themselves to being "established" in a civilized fashion, since they are easily propped against nearby walls, counters, bureaus, sinks, and the like. Their length and the rubber pads at the armpits, handgrips, and tips give them a fighting chance to remain where placed. (Retrieving crutches is just one of countless crutch-life annoyances that need to be recognized and minimized.)

Aluminum underarm crutches: Aluminum crutches are lighter than wooden ones, making them preferable because of the energy they save. Crutching requires much more energy than normal walking, and pointing out ways to conserve strength is a major focus of this book. The design, fitting, and uses of aluminum crutches are identical to those of wood crutches, but the cost will be more.

Elbow, Lofstrand, or Canadian crutches (aluminum only): Canadian crutches require considerably less energy to use, but they are more difficult to master than underarm crutches, and are therefore normally reserved for long-term users or partial-weight-bearing persons. If you have relatively good stability, such crutches may be an option for you after you no longer need to be non–weight-bearing with full length crutches. The strength you save, in addition to faster achievable speeds, are activity-enhancing reasons to make the switch.

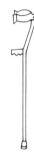

Canadians are designed so that special cuffs keep the crutch attached to your forearm, which permits your hands to be freed for other uses. For proper fit the cuff should extend as high as possible on the forearm without interfering with bending—about one inch below the elbow. Some people feel there is less wrist strain with Canadians than with axillary crutches.

> *Caution:* Canadian crutches extend only to the elbow level. The shorter length and the design make them much less stable, particularly for persons just learning crutch skills. They are not generally advisable for the ambitious, short-term, non-weight-bearing person, who is anxious to "get out and get goin'."

The main drawbacks of Canadian crutches—in addition to stability considerations—is the convenience factor. Because of their shorter length and lack of rubber armpit pads, Canadian crutches are more difficult to establish when you don't need them—retrievals are aggravating and waste energy. For the same reason they are less useful as general-purpose tools than full-length underarm models and, not surprisingly, are almost impossible to use when wearing bulky coats or jackets.

> ***Caution:*** *Never place sleeves of a garment over the arm cuffs.* Additionally, persons who also have neurological conditions may find the arm cuffs themselves a source of entrapment if there is a need to remove them quickly.

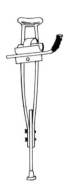

Platform crutches: These crutches are used when weight cannot be taken *through* the forearms or hands, as in combinations of leg injury with an arm fracture or leg injury with arthritis of the hands. To spare the hands, the arms are bent at the elbow, and the weight is taken *on* the forearms, which are clasped and supported on platforms or "gutters." There are grips for the hands. A single platform crutch can be used by one arm in conjunction with an axillary crutch under the other arm. A disadvantage is that you may not be as independent as you'd like, since help is sometimes needed in attaching the arm grips.

Fitting of Crutches

When being fitted for crutches, be wearing the type of shoe that you will be using the most, preferably a flat or low-heeled, rubber-soled sort with good support.

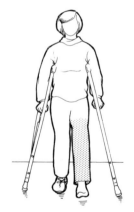

● ● ●Word to the Wise: FITTING. Carefully follow the guidelines below for the correct length of your new acquisitions. All too frequently crutches are fitted improperly—generally too long—even by trained personnel. If underarm crutches are not adjusted correctly, not only will you have extra difficulty in learning to use them, but you may have sore underarms and pinched nerves in the armpit area. Correct fitting results in all your weight being carried on your palms/hands, not in the armpits.

Tripod position: When standing upright the crutch tips should be placed about 10 inches in front of the working foot and 6–10 inches out to the side. The triangle formed by the crutch tips and your good foot provides the maximum stability for a non-weight-bearing person. Body build, strength, and balance will make the dimensions of the tripod slightly different for each person.

Height of crutches: The upper pad (armpit bar) of the crutches should almost reach the armpit, but not touch it, maintaining a space about two inches (two or three fingers) wide between the bar and the armpit. The height is adjusted so your weight is *not* suspended from your armpits.

Handgrips: The handgrips should be placed so that your arms are slightly bent, with elbows flexed at a 20–30-degree angle. (Or, if you let your arms hang relaxed down at your side, the handgrips should be at the level of your wrist crease.) Hands should grip firmly — with confidence.

Arm clench: The crutches will *not* fall out of your armpits — axillae — because you slightly clench your upper arm muscles in toward your body.

Armpit pads: However, do *not* allow the armpit pads to be pressed in tight and hard against the rib cage. (Ouch.) They *will* touch the rib cage, but less pressure means less friction and less soreness.

Posture: Good posture — with your head up and spine straight — is important in avoiding backache or aggravation of any existing back problem. Try to suspend your weight directly over the crutches, attempting to keep them fairly vertical, with the forward lean from the ankle of the good leg.

Lift: Body lift for walking is provided by depression of the shoulders and extension of the elbows.

Injured leg: The leg is held off the ground and carried in front of the body, with the knee bent — or however the leg is casted.

Stability: Placement of the foot is important. In general, and particularly when just learning, the foot is not placed *between* the crutches in any form of non-weight-bearing crutching, because that does not create the safe, three-point tripod position.

Caution: Always *lift* the foot being moved, no matter what gait you are using or what aid you are using. Dragging it or sliding it greatly increases the risk of falling.

Condition of Crutches

Rubber pads: Rubber pads and grips are necessities, not accessories. Do not use crutches without them. If you are borrowing someone else's used crutches, it is highly recommended that you put on new pads unless the originals are in excellent shape — not frayed and broken down. Although there is likely to be some initial tenderness in any case, old soft pads lead to additional soreness in the rib-cage area. Your hands will also get tender, because worn handgrip pads collapse, and the palms will actually be resting on the wood cores. New pads are inexpensive; get them from pharmacies or medical-supply stores.

Crutch tips: If the crutches are secondhand, check the tips to make sure that they are not worn smooth and that no wood is showing through. They should be a minimum of 1½ inches across for maximum stability, with clearly defined, circular grooves in the tread for good traction. Rotating the tips will lengthen their life, and, if available in your area, spikes — which are retractable when not needed — can be attached for winter safety. See Chapter 19 for mail-order information.

Caution: Travel on either ice or snow is not recommended unless absolutely necessary.

Wrist protection: Since there is no padding to protect the wrists from where they rub against the crutch extensions, either wrap the crutches — where needed — with surgical gauze or put small gauze bandages on your wrists until they are toughened up.

Front Edge of Crutches

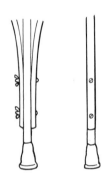

For safety's sake, use your crutches with the rounded flatter head of the adjustable bolts facing front, in the direction you are going — this is the "front edge." The protruding end of the wing nuts on the opposite side of the vertical extensions will, therefore, always be facing toward your back. This prevents the wing nuts from catching on obstacles, draperies, etc., but most important, it keeps them from hooking up on the lips of stair treads when you go up or down stairs — an obscure but very real hazard.

The nuts and bolts of crutches are what make the front and back edges. The bolts are removable in order to adjust the overall height of the crutches and the placement of the handgrips. They can also loosen and fall off. Check them frequently and keep the connections tight.

Expert Moves on Crutches

Establishing crutches: Getting accustomed to traipsing around via crutches also involves getting savvy on how best to keep them handy when you're not using them. It doesn't sound like too monumental a task, but, when you are already frazzled, it can be the last straw when your crutches slither and slide out of reach. The best strategy is to employ the armpit and handgrip pads as contra-slip devices, leaning the crutches against counters, tables, or whatever, in such a way that the rubber, nonslip covers, at either level, are the point of contact.

"Out in the field" and needing to free up one or both hands, with nothing handy to park the crutches against? Prop them against your own body at about waist level.

> *Caution:* Such a ploy will mark you as a true "crutch sophisticate," but be aware that this really is an advanced maneuver. With your weight supported solely on your good leg, your crutch tripod—the position in which the crutches are out to the side and in which you are most stable—has been removed.

Crutch as leg support: When you are sitting down do you need a way to elevate your bum leg? Tuck the armpit end of a crutch under your thigh and perch the injured leg on top. (This gambit also brands you as an old hand in the crutch war.)

Armpit grip: Using underarm crutches requires a technique to free up a hand without always having to establish the crutches against a wall, counter, or the like. Here's how: use your elbow, upper arm, and armpit to trap the crutch tightly against your chest wall, and presto—you've got a free hand. When you've become a crutch expert, you'll even be able to go short distances that way, moving the crutch ahead with shoulder and elbow action while keeping your hand ready to do something useful. See Chapter 14 for more on this technique.

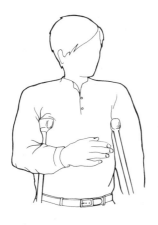 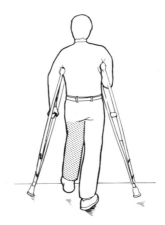

Conservation of Energy

Getting around on crutches is a strenuous form of exercise. Research done by Dr. Robert Waters at the University of Southern California Medical School found that "swing-through" crutching by an exper-

ienced user at a normal speed expends more energy than is used by
unimpaired persons who are walking at their fastest speeds! Average
increase in energy expenditure with crutching is 32 percent, but an
inexperienced fracture patient may have a 69 percent increase in energy
output.

> **Note:** Energy conservation takes careful planning and is a
> major focus of this guide. Heed any tips on how to save, not
> squander, yours.

Basic Crutching: The Beginning "Swing-to" Gait for Non-Weight-Bearing

Less demanding than the swing-to or "swing-through" methods which
follow, this beginning gait is good for anyone weak from surgery or
bed rest, and for those people, especially the elderly, needing a slow and
safe way of walking on crutches with minimum expenditure of energy.
It is almost identical to the advanced swing-to gait—except that the
crutches are moved less ambitiously. One can frequently progress from
this gait to the others.

● ● ●Word to the Wise: GOAL. For persons who are especially weak
from bed rest or who need confidence, having a specific goal a
short distance away, such as a chair where they can rest or a surface
which they can hold on to, is recommended. If a chair is the goal,
turning around and sitting skills should be mastered first. See
Chapter 7.

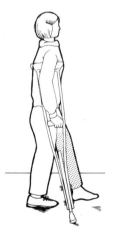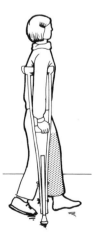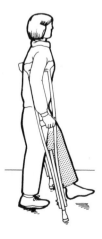

Placement: Place your crutches no more than six inches in front of your good foot. (Longer distances will require you to employ a lot more shoulder strength and expend much more energy.) The disabled leg is held clear of the ground and, if appropriate to your injury, in front of your body.

Step: With stiffened arms and wrists, press against the crutch handles as you lift your good foot up toward—but not all the way to—the placed crutches. Yes, it's slow, s-l-o-w, but you will get there—and that's what counts.

Basic Crutching: The Advanced "Swing-to" Gait for Non-Weight-Bearing

This name refers to the fact that the good leg is stepped or swung just *to* the crutches, and not *through* them, as in more advanced methods. This technique is a good one to start with if you are a beginner in relatively good shape.

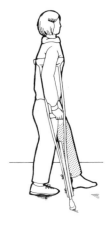

Placement: In a standing position, with your weight on the good leg, place the crutches approximately 10 inches in front of the foot, and 6–10 inches out to either side in the "ready" or "tripod" position.

Step: Stiffen your arms, push down firmly on the handgrips, and push off from your toes, lifting the foot and stepping it forward to a flat landing *just behind* the placed crutches. Your weight will be supported entirely on your hands for a moment before re-placement of the foot.

Re-placement: The crutches, which at that point are barely ahead of your body, will then be placed farther forward of the foot again, in preparation for your next step.

Note: When the crutches are re-placed—established comfortably and securely in front of you—remember that you are under no obligation to keep moving or "swinging-to." There is no need to rush. Until you are sure of yourself and until your strength has improved, this is always the time when you can rest and regroup before continuing.

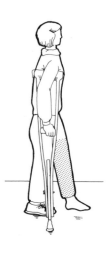

Basic Crutching: The "Swing-through" Gait
for Non-Weight-Bearing

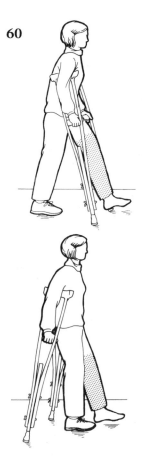

This is the basic workhorse of crutch life and is what you'll be doing after mastering the swing-to. (Be warned, it may also be a *workout*: heart rates can increase anywhere from 60 percent to more than 100 percent over the requirements of normal walking.) The difference from the swing-to is that you swing your body *through* the planted crutches, with the good foot landing in *front* of them—the distance in front being anywhere from 2 to 18 inches, depending upon how experienced you are and how strong and frolicsome you're feeling. (In actuality, the laws of physics make the distance that the foot is placed behind the crutches roughly equal to the distance the foot is naturally swung ahead of the crutches. It's pretty automatic, so you don't have to think much about it.)

Placement: From a standing position, place both crutches about 10 inches in front of you, and 6–10 inches to the side.

Step: Grip the handles firmly, push off from your toes, swing your body forward—weight momentarily supported entirely on your hands—and land heel first on the good foot in front. The crutches will remain momentarily behind your body, but your weight will be concentrated on the planted foot. The crutches will then be swung forward once more to the tripod position.

Caution: Your instinct, undoubtedly, will be to be conservative at first, but let's make it official: take small steps, look where you are going, and check out the terrain before moving.

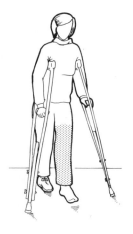

Note: If you need to take a break, hang out just like that by remaining in the tripod position for awhile. (When your balance is better and your muscles stronger, you might occasionally forsake this professionally endorsed "R and R" position for the alternative of simply placing your crutches out to the sides.) Take a break, and when ready, continue trekking by swinging through again. That's really all there is to this workhorse variety of walking on crutches.

Besides the obvious options of sitting down or sacking out—and the obvious observation that furniture for such options is not always available—knowing other ways to rest is vital for those on crutches. Not a moment should be lost in acquiring the tricks of *this* trade.

Wall winner: This can be employed wherever there is a sturdy, head-height, vertical surface by simply changing direction and backing yourself against the chosen surface. Divvy up your body weight between your back—against the wall—and your good leg and foot. The crutches support a little weight too. It's simple, and can be used anywhere: in your home, a museum, an elevator—or against a handy tree.

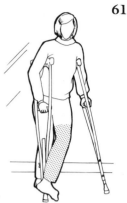

Crutch catch: This is a way to rest the hard-working muscles which keep your injured leg and its cast off the ground. Wherever you are—plane, train, or Spain—just establish yourself and your crutches in a sturdy tripod position, then lay the weighty leg, the useless one, over the strong-side crutch opposite to it. Hang out there and relax. Needless to point out, the crutch catch can be combined with the wall winner.

Foot frenzy: Obvious to one and all, the good foot takes a major beating doing all that work by itself. It's hard to really rest it without the aforementioned furniture, but a certain amount of relief can be provided simply by rocking back and forth between the heel and toe. Can be done anywhere—including on the sidelines of your son's soccer game—in addition to being combined with wall winners and crutch catches.

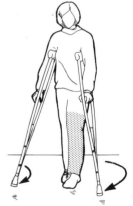

Basic Crutching: Change of Direction for Non-Weight-Bearing

Positioning: Assume the tripod position, weight on good foot and crutches properly placed.

Placement: Move the crutch tips a few inches in the direction you wish to turn. It is safest to turn in the direction of your good leg.

Step: Step to the crutches. Repeat until you are turned in the direction you wish to go.

Mastered that? Below are more advanced techniques that will help you get around with improved safety, conservation of energy, and—when you're ready for it—a lot more pizzaz and speed.

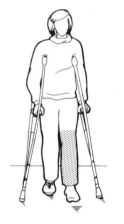

Advanced Crutching: Change of Direction for Non-Weight-Bearing

You've got to have the option to turn and go in other directions, and there's an easier way than hopping around like an ungainly stork. Here's a smooth alternative.

Positioning: Assume the tripod position, weight on good foot, hands and crutches in place—ahead and to the side, wherever you've learned to prefer them.

Shoulder turn: Turn both shoulders and swing both crutches in the direction you wish to go, and at the same instant—

Foot pivot: Shift most of your weight to the ball of your foot, then pivot on it in the same direction as the crutches.

Presto. There you are—turned around—and possibly feeling pretty proud of yourself.

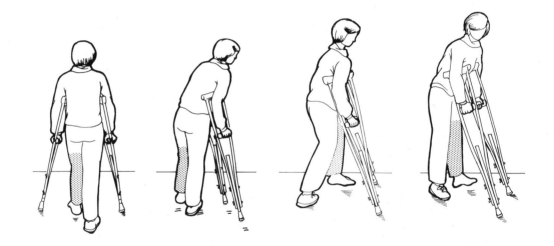

Advanced Crutching: Sideways Movement for Non-Weight-Bearing

There are plenty of occasions when you need to get through narrow spaces — maybe congestion at the local mall or crowded aisles in a plane or at the office. No problem—read on.

Turn: Change direction, or pivot (see above) so you are sideways to the space you want to pass through.

Positioning: Bring the crutch of your choice in close to your body, right next to your hip.

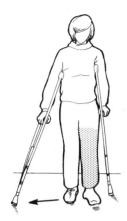
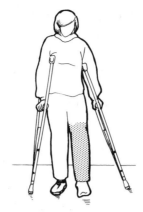

Placement: Extend the other crutch a comfortable distance in the direction you are sidling, and hop next to it with your trusty and sturdy uninjured leg.

Keep going: Repeat, bringing the first crutch close once more and so on. As you see, no problem, which is lucky—as you'll be using these moves a lot.

Caution: This is an advanced maneuver, requiring good balance, because at this point you have abandoned the stability of the tripod position.

Advanced Crutching: Crutch Swing for Non-Weight-Bearing

Instead of swinging your crutches directly straight ahead and parallel to your sides, try swinging them forward in an arc away from your body. This slightly circular swing saves energy because your body weight need not be raised so high off the ground to accommodate the length of the crutches. The wider swing also allows increased tolerance for

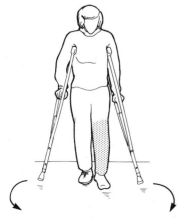
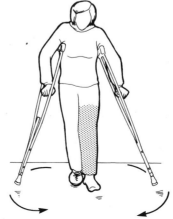

rough surfaces and other protruding hazards that might trip you up. Since you are an advanced dude when you do this, you will have already figured out that use of this more expansive swing is mostly restricted to wide-open places and spaces.

Advanced Crutching: Power Crutching for Non-Weight-Bearing

Ready to be speedier and sportier, wanting a workout, or trying to feel athletic again after all you've been through? To get more bounce to the ounce, use your now oh-so-powerful good leg in a more forceful fashion. Power crutching, in conjunction with the arced crutch swing described above, makes one dynamic duo.

Step: From the tripod position as you swing your good leg through, land on your *heel*—not the full, flat foot—with the knee flexed.

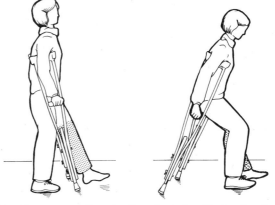

Heel roll-off: Immediately "explode" off the heel, rolling your weight onto the toes by straightening the leg.

Toe push-off: Then push off strongly from the toes themselves. You should be able to feel those calf muscles and toes work.

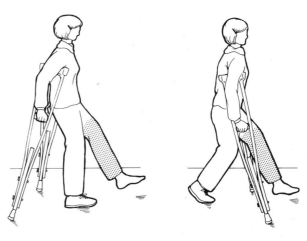

Landing: Now swing your leg forward through the placed crutches as far ahead as your sense of adventure, fun, and balance will allow.

So to recap—it's land on your heel with the knee flexed, quickly push off the heel on to your toes by straightening the leg, then a final forceful fling from the toes themselves. This spine-tingling technique will add a whole new dimension to your crutch life, but for safety's sake—because of the buildup in speed—is recommended only on level or uphill terrain.

Now, get out on your driveway, street, or lawn and let "power crutching" raise your spirits as well as your metabolism—not to mention amazing your family and neighbors.

HILLS, INCLINES, RAMPS, CITY STREETS, CURBS, AND UNFAMILIAR TERRAIN

Ascents

Power-crutching techniques are the way to go with steep hills, since the powerful leg extension gives you the push-up you require.

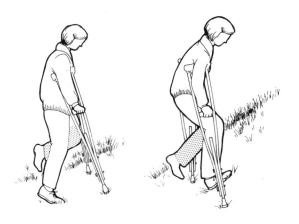

Descents

Crutches at the ready: Your elbows will be heavily bent, with the crutches at such an angle that they ressemble a pair of pistols you've pulled out of a hip holster.

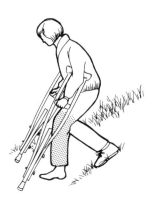

Heel strike: Because of the steep slope, the heel will land close to the crutches, rather than ahead of them (the normal way for advanced crutching on the flat).

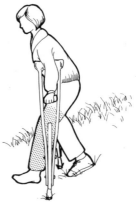

Knee bend: Bend your knee deeply going down hills, landing each time on your heel, the crutches well out in front, at about a 45-degree angle to the slope.

Heel roll: Once the heel has been placed under a well-flexed knee and leg, you roll the weight onto the whole foot.

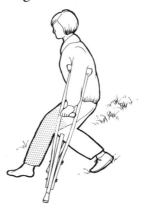

What do you think? Are you inspired to get out of the house and try a few daring moves?

Crossing Streets

By the time you're crossing streets, you'll have an established and confident career in assistive aids of any kind—and will know that basically what is required in city scampering is good judgment and good timing.

Watch the traffic lights: Observe the cycle of the traffic lights and traffic for a couple of minutes.

Cross with traffic lights: If available, *always.*

Cross with others: Plan to cross with others if you feel there is safety in numbers.

Stay visible: However, don't get in a crowd where your slower pace and mobility aid(s) can be overlooked.

Get help: Ask someone to accompany you if you feel there is the slightest chance that there is inadequate time available to get across.

Ready, set, go: Above all, *be prepared.* When the light changes or the slack in traffic appears, get going.

Unfamiliar Terrain

Take it easy when you're going anywhere new. If you're in a field or on a strange lawn, there may be soft spots that might trap a crutch tip, hidden indentations, slippery stones, or a stick which could roll from under your crutch. In the city, there are uneven sidewalks and pot holes in the streets. At a strange house, there are the hazards of rugs, slippery floors, different stairs, and the like. *Don't take anything for granted until you are thoroughly familiar with your surroundings.*

PARTIAL-WEIGHT-BEARING WITH CRUTCHES

Being allowed to place weight on your injured limb after weeks or months of treating it both like a distant relative *and* like a beloved and thoroughly spoiled offspring, is an occasion most people don't forget. For those recovering from fractures, weight-bearing is especially good news because it stimulates bone growth at the site of the break. For everyone else, it will halt bone loss due to lack of use.

The partial-weight-bearing stage may last quite a while or just a few days. In almost every case, walking will seem strange no matter how you do it or what assistive device you use to ease the transition. A few points to ponder follow.

• • •Word to the Wise: STAGES. Passing through the stages of partial-weight-bearing — using both crutches to start with, then a single crutch, and finally a cane — may make you feel you're babying yourself or being a wimp. Not true. Progressing from one device to another, each requiring more participation of the recovering leg, means that the muscles are building up and the resulting gait is returning to normal.

Another way to rebuild and perfect walking skills is in the shallow end of a swimming pool, where the water itself acts as the assistive aid and allows your hands to be swung freely.

Note: If you're starting your crutch career at this level rather than at the non-weight-bearing stage, read the appropriate entries at the beginning of this chapter for selection and measurement of crutches, in addition to other essential information.

Note: If canes or a walker are prescribed for your partial-weight-bearing stage, see Chapter 6.

General Guidelines for Partial-Weight-Bearing

Level surfaces: The injured or weak leg or foot always steps first.

Ascending stairs and curbs: The good leg or foot always steps up first.

Descending stairs and curbs: The injured leg or foot always steps down first.

Note: The subject of stairs will be treated at length in Chapter 8.

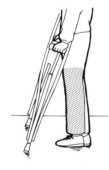

The "Step-to" Gait for Partial-Weight-Bearing

This name refers to the fact that the injured leg is stepped *to* the crutches, and the good leg is brought up next to it.

Positioning: In a standing position, with your weight mostly on the healthy leg and the proper (prescribed) percentage of weight on your injured leg, place the crutches approximately 10 inches in front of your feet, and 6–10 inches out to either side in the tripod position.

Note: Generally, your doctor will prescribe how much weight should be put on the recovering leg. If possible, step on a scale with your injured leg to get a feel of how much that weight is.

Step: Using the crutches as partial support, step the injured leg forward in as natural a way as possible, placing the heel and then the whole foot just behind the crutches. Try to have the correct amount of weight bearing on it.

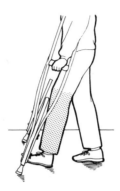

Best foot forward: Bring the good foot and leg up next to it. The crutches, which at that point are in line with your body, will then be brought forward in front again, in preparation for your next step.

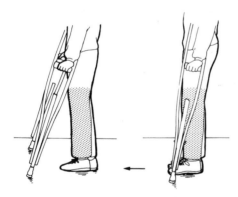

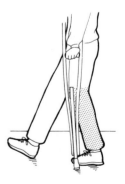

The "Step-through" Gait for Partial-Weight-Bearing

This name refers to the fact that the injured leg is stepped to the crutches, and the good leg then steps *through* past the injured leg, a pattern that develops normal walking. By this time you may be putting equal weight on both legs — but because your injured leg is weak, substantial support is still needed. The technique is similar to the step-to gait, except that the step is longer and therefore closer to normal walking.

"Four-Point Gait" for Partial-Weight-Bearing

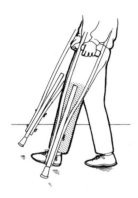

You may start off with this advanced gait, or you may have to work up to it, but it's a big step closer to normal walking. You no longer move the crutches first, then step the weak leg and finally the good one. Change to simultaneously picking up both crutches and advancing the weak leg. The foot-step and placement of the crutches will be simultaneous and for an equal distance. Three points of the four-point gait are now established and stable; the fourth point, the strong leg, moves forward alone.

● ● ●Word to the Wise: HEEL STRIKE. Wherever you are practicing, and with whatever device, always try to achieve heel strike (heel hitting the ground first) and as normal a gait as possible. Abnormal gait means imbalance, strain of other muscles or joints, and *slower* progress to full recovery.

Recovering with Walker, Cane, or Wheelchair   6

Assistive aids are generally prescribed on the basis of type of injury, the extent of support the devices provide, how stable they are, the degree of energy expenditure and coordination required to use them, plus the person's overall fitness. One individual with a leg fracture may be able to use crutches, while another with an identical injury will be safer and more mobile with a walker.

Mobility aids make getting out of bed possible, probably their most crucial function. Standing up on your feet compels physical systems to fight—to their benefit—against the pull of gravity, forcing muscles to contract and creating pressure throughout the body. Legs and ankles don't swell so much, bones don't lose so much calcium, and food is more likely to pass properly and easily through the digestive tract.

Paradoxically, staying in bed is tiring. Thanks to that restful position, breathing is not as efficient, oxygen doesn't get dispersed, and systems are not "on go." Even the cells and antibodies which protect against infection become lazy. No one needs that! Mobility aids free you from the perils of bed rest. Bed rest—in most cases—is *too* restful for good health.

As strength and abilities increase, persons often progress from one assistive device to another, from the most support to the least—using any or all of the following in some combination: walker to underarm (axillary) crutches, elbow (Canadian) crutches, broad-based canes, and finally, regular single-based canes.

It can be a distressing process to acknowledge loss of function. Sometimes there is reluctance—or actual refusal—to use mobility devices. Whether it is because they represent visible signs of disability, or because of fear of being dependent on them, such refusal can mean loss of opportunity. Mobility aids expand the scope of possible activities and promote safety in doing so. They help in reducing the pain of movement that leads to a sedentary lifestyle and the vicious circle of deconditioning, less flexibility, more pain, and more restriction. *Canes, walkers and wheelchairs are tools to let you live life more fully.*

Whether you are purchasing, renting or borrowing a mobility aid, it is advisable to check with your doctor or physical therapist concerning its suitability, safety, ease of use, and cost. An aid which gives your body more support than it should have will hinder muscular recovery.

> *Caution:* Frequent falls suggest that the proper device is not being used or that you need additional training with that particular device.

● ● ●Word to the Wise: GOAL. For those who are especially weak from bed rest or who need confidence, having a specific goal a short distance away, such as a chair where they can rest or a counter which they can hold on to, is recommended. If a chair is the goal, turning around and sitting skills should be mastered first. See Chapter 7 for more on sitting.

WALKER

Walkers are the most stable of the mobility aids, followed by underarm crutches, Canadian crutches, two canes and lastly, the single cane. Walkers demand the least coordination, requiring the user only to pick up and move a three-sided tubular frame, and then walk into it. Their drawback is their shape, which, unlike crutches, prohibits any serious innovation or improvisation — not to mention frolicsome footwork or speed.

Types of Walkers

Walkers come in many styles and are selected according to disability and considerations such as balance, coordination, and strength. Get advice from a professional before buying.

Pick-up walker (without wheels): Although walkers without wheels require lifting, they are sufficiently stable for most people and can theoretically be used in ascending stairs if the width of their bases is narrow enough (but see below for more on stairs). This type is the least expensive.

Rolling walker, optional brakes: Usually wheels are only on the front legs, with or without brakes. "Gutters" or platforms can be added for persons with simultaneous arm and leg injuries. Rolling walkers allow constant contact with the ground and can be more stable for some people, particularly those who are too weak to pick up a walker. Wheeled walkers cannot be used on stairs.

> *Caution:* Brakeless wheeled walkers can roll away from a person and are hazardous for those with poor balance, co-ordination, or judgment. However, sophisticated brake systems are now available, including one which automatically locks when a person is leaning on the walker.

Reciprocal walker: A specialized walker that allows a normal pattern of leg movement for a person with good balance. It is used for "gait training" — or learning to walk correctly again, by those who are newly ambulatory after an extended non-weight-bearing regimen. Sometimes persons with walking casts use such walkers to help maintain correct gait. Elderly persons may find them difficult to use.

Options for Walkers

Height: The height must be adjustable; extensions are available for the extra-tall.

Width: The width of a walker refers to the tubular arms and to the base. The angle of the upright bars influences the amount of stability and support.

Weight: Aluminum lightweight walkers are suitable for most people; a sturdier grade of tubing is recommended for heavier individuals. Wheeled models — because of terrain demands — generally are of heavier construction.

Portability: Walkers should be collapsible in order to be put into a car or to be placed out of the way in restaurants, the workplace, and elsewhere.

Forearm supports and crutch extensions: Additions such as these are available to provide underarm support for patients with combination arm and leg injuries or persons without the strength to keep their weight on their hands.

Other modifications: Carry-all baskets, seats for resting, cane clips, and oversize wheels for "fun and games" outside are sophisticated additions that add convenience and cost. The *apron* — invaluable, recommended, and described in Chapter 14 — will handle many of your toting chores, but a simple pouch or caddy to hang on a walker is

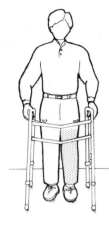

probably worth the investment. See Chapter 19 for obtaining walker modifications.

Fitting of Walkers

Wear suitable shoes, and then adjust the walker so that the handlebars come to the level of your wrist crease. You should be able to stand up straight *without* hunching the shoulders when you put your weight on the frame.

Techniques for Walkers

Pick-up walkers: You have two choices. Advance the walker first, and then step into it with — if possible — each leg taking an equal step.

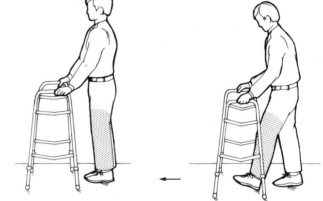

Or advance the walker and simultaneously step with one foot, advance it again and simultaneously step with the other foot.

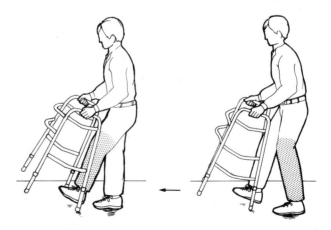

> *Note:* Try to achieve "heel strike"—placing the heel first—and as normal a walking gait as possible.

Which leg to use first: The person who is partial-weight-bearing—who is not yet allowed to put full weight on the recovering limb, steps in with the injured leg first. (The only exception is in ascending stairs, when the weaker leg goes first.)

Turning: Use small steps to rotate, turning the walker in the direction of the stronger leg.

Sitting: Again using small, safe steps, turn around with your walker in front of the chair, bed, or whatever. Back up until you feel the chair against the back of your legs. Reach back for the arm rests or seat, be sure you are centered, and sit. For a complete countdown on sitting, see Chapter 7.

Stairs: In theory there are walkers that are designed for stairs, but in reality—if a person is able to handle stairs at all—a handrail should be used on one side and a cane (a small quad-based cane) or crutch on the other. If you are going to be using a walker for a long time, have one walker at the top of the stairs and another one at the bottom so wherever you arrive, top or bottom, there is a way to continue.

Non-weight-bearing: A walker can be used instead of crutches for keeping a limb off the ground. Generally, however, this is not practical unless the non-weight-bearing period of time is extremely short, the distance to be covered minimal, or one's physical status indicates use of a walker will be more successful than use of crutches. In such a case, the walker is moved while the individual hops up to and in it on the supporting leg. Good balance is required.

Precautions for Walkers

Folded walker: If a walker has been folded and then unfolded and set up for use, be sure the legs are fully and securely snapped into place before supporting yourself on it.

Standing up: When rising from a seated position, do not pull yourself up on the walker. Scoot forward to the edge of your seat, and bring your feet under your body so that your weight will be centered over them. Keep your feet separated to improve stability, and brace the backs of your knees or legs against the chair. Lean forward slightly, and push up from the armrests or seating surface instead of from the walker.

> *Note:* When attempting to stand up, you may find that having your feet one in front of the other in a short-stride position is easier than when they are parallel.

Moving the walker: Lift the walker with both hands, and put all four legs down at the same time. Placement of back and front legs separately is less stable.

Front bar: For maximum stability, advance in the walker to about six inches of the front bar. Do *not* lean against it.

Ramps: Be careful, especially going down, because the grade slants away from you and balance is tricky.

CANE

Not so long ago the "walking stick" was an essential part of a fashionable man's wardrobe — to be twirled and twiddled — to impart impressive dash and swagger. Nowadays the cane is strictly a helpmate, and pretty much taken for granted. No professional is hovering around to make sure you get the correct one, as with crutches or wheelchairs. Canes frequently just "happen" — borrowed, retrieved from an attic, or rescued from a relative — lowly, little-understood, and very likely pretty ineffectual due to simple lack of knowledge. Canes, however, are not the pushovers they appear to be; most people do not use them efficiently or properly. Using a cane shows wisdom — and using one correctly will get you back to normal, faster — equally balanced — in two-legged weight-bearing.

Function of Canes

The cane really is a helpmate, as you will see from all the wonderful ways it can assist you: it is truly underrated, underappreciated, and underused.

Weight-bearing and "unloading":   Although canes do not support a lot of weight, even a small load relief can make walking a possiblity for many people.

Stability: A cane's major reason for existing.

Propulsion: Canes deliver about one-fifth the propulsive force of a healthy leg.

● ● ●Word to the Wise: SPEED. Don't be overly hasty with your newly acquired "cane craft." The *amount of time* a cane is in contact with the floor helps impart the propulsion.

Promotion of normal gait: Canes, innocuous as they may seem, fill a crucial void in the recovery of a person who no longer needs crutches—fostering *correct* gait patterns as a person returns to normal, two-legged walking. Limping, which is abnormal gait that can produce strain and fatigue throughout the body, is minimized, while good walking habits are practiced from the beginning. Your posture should be upright and not leaning out over the cane.

Cane as a warning signal: Another reason to carry a cane is that—particularly in crowded and bustling areas, such as airports, metropolitan streets, or transportation systems—it is a warning to passersby that you do not move well, normally, or quickly.

Caution: Be aware that four-legged (quad) canes can be hazardous to *other* persons because of their large bases.

Cane as a tool: Don't let your cane languish. Use it with flair and flourish—to reach, to pull, to push, to pound (if really frustrated), to persuade (a threat of a caning will be all that's ever needed), and eventually, when recovery and rehabilitation are over and done with—to pirouette.

Types of Canes

The field of assistive devices has seen enormous progress in recent years, thanks to new materials and technologies as well as increased attention to the needs of the mobility challenged. Read on for revelations about canes.

J-line cane: The basic ("normal") standby—either wood or aluminum—but no longer necessarily the best choice.

Swan-neck cane: This preferred design places the user's weight directly over the tip when the cane is in contact with the floor—making it both more stable and energy efficient. The swan-neck cane is always made of aluminum; its light weight makes it suitable for individuals of all strength levels in terms of energy required and energy expended.

Quad cane: Multipoint canes are mainly for balance and come with small or large bases. Besides offering the best stability, they are agreeable in that they stay upright when a person lets go of them.

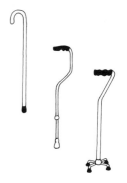

However, on the road back to normal walking, quads are only an intermediate step—with a single-tipped cane the goal. Ultimately, the single-tip is preferable since it promotes increased strength and standard gait.

Collapsible cane: This kind folds up so it can be carried in a purse or bag, handy for the occasional user. See Chapter 19 for where to obtain a collapsible cane.

Materials Used for Canes

Wooden ones have the character, but aluminum canes are lighter and have advantageous designs.

Handles of Canes

Types: A flat "T-handle" is frequently preferable to a curved one, which does not distribute weight but concentrates it on a small part of the palm.

Size: The size of a handle is important too. Large hands—or arthritic hands with reduced grasping capability—need larger handles. Foam padding taped to the handle is one solution.

Transporting canes: Canes with curved handles can be hooked in a belt, trouser pocket, or shirt front or dangled from the crook of your flexed arm. They can be suspended on a drawer, arm of a chair, or shower-curtain rod. Alas, the efficient, flat (T-handled) canes are not so adaptable. Remember, the quad canes don't fall at all.

Fitting of Canes

Measuring for a cane is similar to that for walkers, requiring that you wear nonslip, supportive shoes and select a cane whose handle aligns with the crease of your wrist when your arm is hanging loosely at your side.

> *Note:* Two-thirds of the people who buy canes get one that is too long—affecting its potential for support, propulsion, and gait retraining. Twenty percent get them too short. Be different, join the minority: get a unique, one-of-a-kind cane if you wish but have it the correct length. Wooden canes can be cut; aluminum models are adjustable.

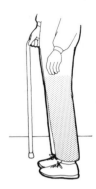

Using a cane, which appears so simple and basic, actually poses a dilemma for many users—*which* hand carries the cane?

Which hand: The hand which carries the cane usually is the one *opposite* to your disabled side. In normal walking, the *opposite* arm and leg move together; using a cane duplicates that customary pattern: the weak leg is paired with the cane being carried on the opposite (stronger) side. Stability is enhanced not only by the balancing of weak with strong but in the creation of a longer stride. (A short stride is considered a risk factor for falls.)

Beginning walking: When you are first getting reaccustomed to walking or when you're dealing with a noticeably weaker leg, start out by moving your cane forward first, then advance the weak foot so that its toes are on a level with the cane, and finally bring up the stronger leg. Keep the cane fairly close for stability.

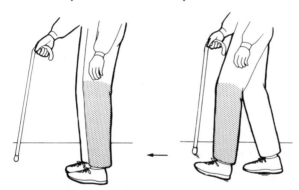

Advanced walking: You will progress to moving the weak leg and the cane at the same time. Remember, the cane stays in the opposite hand to the weak leg. Try to achieve as normal a walk as possible, including "heel strike"—placing the heel first.

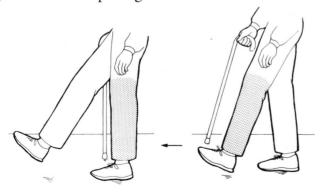

Ascending stairs: As it will be doing the work of raising the body weight, remind yourself "good leg first" and step up with it. Use the cane for support in your strong-side hand as you step. Next lift the injured leg to the same stair, and lastly, bring the cane up. If there's a railing, grab it for additional support if needed, or use it to help pull yourself up. Even a plain wall may help with balance. Slow and tedious, to be sure, but you'll soon be stronger, and who knows—maybe taking stairs two at a time before long. For additional help on stairs, see Chapter 8.

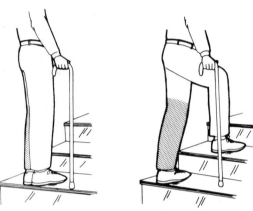

Note: If, owing to previous injury, your "strong" leg isn't that strong, and you have difficulty going up stairs with a single-tip cane, consider using the more supportive quad cane or a single underarm crutch. The latter will allow increased lift-up since shoulder strength is employed. You might leave one of these critters parked at the stairs for whenever help is needed.

In situations of extreme weakness or multiple injury, a railing is essential—but sometimes it's on the wrong side for your particular need. The solution, an "ultra" one (but who cares?), is to go up backward—presto, the railing is on the side where it can help.

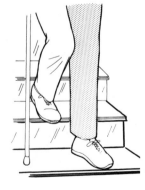

Descending stairs: Think "bad leg first." Place the toes of your good foot so that they overlap the edge of the step and get you closer to "take-off." Hold on to the railing or wall if necessary, and step down with the injured limb. When firmly established, step down with the other leg.

> *Caution:* As in ascending, you can get the railing on the needed side by going down backward, but balance and spatial judgment must be very good. Backing up or down stairs is not particularly recommended, but the techniques are included to encourage adaptability and perseverance in achieving independence.

Standing up: Scoot forward to the edge of your seat, and bring your feet under your body so your weight will be centered over them. Keep your feet separated to improve stability, and brace the backs of your knees or legs against the chair. Lean forward slightly, and push up from the armrests or the seating surface. You can have the cane in your hand, but use the armrests to push up on.

● ● ●Word to the Wise: FEET. You may find that positioning your feet one in front of the other in a short-stride position when trying to stand up is easier than when they are parallel.

Curbs: Curbs are handled like steps, but here's a quick recap. *Ascending.* Step up onto the sidewalk with your strong foot, while pushing off with the cane and transfering your weight to that strong leg. *Descending.* When stepping off a curb, position yourself at the edge and place the cane onto the street. Step down with the weak leg. When that leg is stable, with the knee straight and supporting your weight, step down with the strong foot.

Partial-weight-bearing with two canes: Rather than two crutches, two canes may be your ticket to get walking once more. At the beginning, as with partial-weight-bearing using crutches, the canes are advanced first, then the weak leg, and finally the strong leg. Similarly, as strength improves, the canes and weak leg are moved simultaneously, with the better leg last. (See Chapter 5, "Four-Point Gait.")

Which hand? (Exception due to pain):   Experts suggest that the exception to carrying the cane in the hand opposite the involved leg is in cases of severe disability or pain. Such a situation takes precedence over gait retraining, prevention of muscle strain, and other considerations. Realistically, however, in such cases a walker or crutches should be employed instead of a cane.

Wintertime safety: Metal ice-gripping cane tips are available. A ski pole of the proper height is a practical alternative.

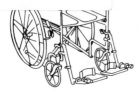

WHEELCHAIR

When appropriate, a wheelchair may offer *more* activity and maintain a wider range of activities than canes, walkers, or crutches. If, during the early phase of your recovery, you have had extended bed rest, have multiple extremity injuries, or are generally out of condition, temporarily renting a wheelchair may be worth considering while you are gaining strength and learning to use your crutches. As a tool to live life more fully, a wheelchair can enhance safety, independence (getting to the bathroom, for instance), and participation in your business and family life. Part-time and temporary full-time use of a wheelchair saves energy for other goals.

● ● ●Word to the Wise: LIBERATION. Do not commit the common error of considering wheelchair use as being "confined." "Confined" is relative—in your case, and most every other case, think "liberated"—for all sorts of jobs and joys.

Function: Conservation of Energy

A wheelchair is a wise choice for elderly persons recovering from leg injury or hip replacement, whose aerobic capacity may no longer be up to the demands of crutches. Use of a wheelchair for longer distances—by anyone—can save energy for the activity contemplated at the destination.

> *Note:* It is a common misperception that persons in wheelchairs are paralyzed. The majority of users employ wheelchairs to conserve energy, either because of injury, age, or neurological conditions.

Options for Wheelchairs

Except for permanent use, wheelchairs are usually rented and do not need meticulous fitting. The standard issue prescribed by physical therapists for orthopaedic patients is sturdy, simple, and relatively inexpensive. However, there are options that definitely make you more comfortable and independent—so check them out below.

Weight of chair: Wheelchairs have benefited greatly from development of aerospace materials, but standard models are still fairly heavy. If you have good balance, rent the lightest possible. "Sports chairs" are in that category but are generally not available for rental.

Armrests: Removable armrests which permit a wheelchair to be moved in close to a table or desk are a highly recommended convenience. They are a necessity if both legs are injured, because they allow you to exit the chair sideways. Lastly, if you are planning to lift a wheelchair in and out of a car, the chair is lighter to load with the armrests removed.

Footrests: Footrests come in several sizes, and should have heel loops to keep the foot from sliding back under the wheelchair. Footrest plates are swung away or turned to the side for exiting, and are removable. If you are using a wheelchair in combination with crutches, bring the crutches along by placing the paired tips on the footrest of your good-side leg and wedging the long part between your hip and the armrest. If your wheelchair is being pushed, stand the crutches upright on the footrest.

Leg rests: "Swing-away" leg and foot rests both provide extra room for standing up, and are particularly helpful if you are establishing yourself on crutches. An elevating leg rest is mandatory if swelling is a consideration or if you have a rigid, full-length cast or brace. If you will be taking the wheelchair anywhere, leg rests should be removable, since they add considerable length as well as weight.

Collapsible wheelchair: The standard chair is folded by raising the foot plates, placing your hand under the seat, and pulling up. Most people choose a folding model so that they can get into wheels of *another* kind—either your own or someone else's car—for reasons of work, entertainment, or both.

Seat cushion: A cushion is crucial, since sitting for long periods can not only be very uncomfortable but actually lead to tissue breakdown (pressure sores). However, if a wheelchair is not going to be a part of your life for long or is used part-time, an ordinary cushion will do; specialized cushions can be costly. Walking of any kind, even just standing, will stave off sores and keep your backside brawny.

Caution: Pressure relief for the buttocks, every 10–15 minutes, is a must for persons in wheelchairs who are unable to walk at all. Besides the obvious wriggle-and-wiggle method to raise each buttock alternately, "sitting push-ups" are the method of choice, as follows.

Your chair must be in the locked position, your hands on the armrests. Pushing down on your hands, straighten your arms while extending your head and neck upward and

---

depressing your shoulders. Contract your abdominal muscles, tuck your buttocks in, and raise yourself off the seat. Depending upon your strength your legs may rest or be raised horizontally on the seat. Don't forget to breathe naturally. See also Chapter 3. (Sounds like a crazy push-up, but it does do the trick—the premise being "not to let your backside down by lifting it up.") And, hey, you're working those crucial arm muscles at the same time.

Sizes of Wheelchairs

Although exact measurements are not necessary for the short-term user, there are different sizes available that determine what will be most comfortable.

Width: Youth: 14 inches
Narrow Adult: 16 inches
Standard Adult: 18 inches
Wide Adult: 19 or 20 inches

There should be a space of about an inch between the armrest and the hips on each side.

Note: When in doubt, go for the narrower chair, as it will let you get through more doorways, one of the major barriers to wheelchair independence.

Seat depth and back height: These are generally standard unless especially ordered.

Footrest length: Length is adjustable on all chairs.

• • ●Word to the Wise: FOOTREST LENGTH. It is very important that the foot plates be set so that your knees are the same height as, or just *lower* than, your hips. This adjustment is for stability and to keep excessive pressure off the "ischial tuberosities"—the intriguingly named bony protuberances of your backside. "Long-termers" fear pressure sores, and you want to avoid them also.

"Hemi" wheelchair: This chair has other specialized uses but is particularly suitable for orthopaedic patients who are very short—those under five feet—since the design places it closer to the ground. Standing is safer and easier because such individuals' legs can then reach the floor.

• • •Word to the Wise: WHEELCHAIR OPTIONS. Be sure *you* (as well as anyone accompanying you) know how to operate the equipment on your wheelchair *before* you wheel off with it. A lot of aggravation will be saved at a time when you most want to avoid it.

Techniques for Wheelchairs

> *Caution: The point to remember, and it's crucial, is that the wheelchair brakes must be in a locked position any time you wish to stand up or sit down in it.* The safest method is to get into the habit of locking them every time you stop your momentum. In addition, you will want to remember to move the footrests aside before standing and to watch out for your fingers when going through narrow doorways.

Standing up: Lock your chair, and place the footrests to the side. Scoot forward to the edge of your seat, and if you are non-weight-bearing, bring your working foot under your body so your weight will be centered over it. Improve stability by bracing the back of your knee or leg against the chair. Lean forward slightly, and push up from the armrests. See Chapter 7 for more help on standing and sitting.

• • •Word to the Wise: FEET. If you are able to put weight on both legs, you may find that having your feet one in front of the other in a short-stride position when you stand up is easier than standing with the feet parallel.

Sitting: Be sure the chair is locked and the footrests swung aside. Turn around and back up until you feel the chair against the rear of your leg(s). Reach back for the armrests or seat. Hold on, be sure you are centered, and sit.

Doors: Various ways of simplifying doors are to tie them open, wedge them open, and in the case of doorways that are too narrow — to temporarily remove the doors. Bathroom doors generally cause the most problems; they are generally narrow because builders and architects do not have to allow extra space for the passage of large pieces of furniture.

7   Sitting Down and Standing Up Made Easy

Compared to a lot of techniques you'll be introduced to, standing and sitting are relatively uncomplicated. But even such seemingly simple and taken-for-granted procedures will be difficult if you are weak from recent surgery or bed rest. Consider how many times you stand up or sit down in the course of a day, and you'll soon see that an easier way will save you tons of energy—and the *right* way may save you a fall or two.

The skills which follow will not only enable you to adapt quickly to life at home and on the job, but will also provide solutions to problems in other settings. The more challenging maneuvers may never be needed, but they are included to provide impetus and incentive to try—on any level—to attain independence for yourself and those around you.

> *Caution:* For the non-weight-bearing or partially-weight-bearing person with crutches, the key to safe sitting is to have your good leg touching the chair, sofa, bed—or whatever you are planning to park yourself on—*before* you make the actual move to sit. Since your leg is pressed against a solid, stationary object, *you* are solid and stable also—and you are assured that whatever you are planning to sit on is indeed right there.

Basic Sitting Down

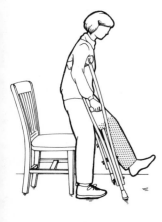

Positioning: Place yourself close to the chair (bed, couch, stool, or whatever) and turn around (see Chapter 5).

Chair touch: Hop back a pace so that the calf of your good leg is *pressed* against the chosen spot. Be sure you are centered. (If the chair is fragile or movable in any way, just touch with your calf. Do not press hard.)

Lowering: Remove the crutches from your armpits, pair them, and with your strong-side hand hold them by the near wooden extensions. Use them for balance in that hand, and with the other hand reach back to hold on to the seat as you sit.

(Professionals recommend holding the crutches on the injured-leg side, but muscular strength and control by the supporting leg is better utilized if you hold them on your strong side. Your choice.)

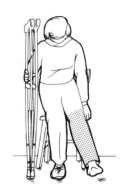

Note: An optional method is sliding both hands from the handgrips to the *forward* wooden extensions, so that the crutches have been removed from the armpit to stand vertical and directly in front of you. (Do not pair them.) With one crutch in each hand balance yourself with their support, bend your good leg, and sit down. This is a more advanced technique since you are not holding on to the chair with either hand. Be sure the chair is stable and that you are centered.

• • ●Word to the Wise: ESTABLISHING CRUTCHES. Friends, relatives, associates, and acquaintances—all will hasten to put your crutches nicely aside for you. Be polite but be savvy and self-reliant—stand or lay them next to your chair. Then they're yours when you need them.

Sitting Down, Standing Up: Sophisticated Moves

Chair-touch: The crutch sophisticate will execute the chair-touch so that the calf is pressing or touching at an *angle,* not straight on. Although seemingly trivial, in actuality the angled leg prevents the chair from being pushed away from you by the bulge of your calf muscles as you sit down.

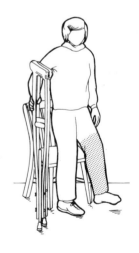

Improved view: An angled chair-touch sets up a much safer execution, the angled approach giving a better view of where your posterior is heading and a better chance of centering yourself. Definitely preferable to plopping down with only a prayer that the *chair seat* is where it should be.

Cramped approach: In a crowded setting, such as a restaurant, it sometimes helps to push the chair itself on an angle, so you have enough space to perform the angled touch.

Reclining chair: If you expect to be out of commission for a long time with a need to keep an ankle, knee, or foot elevated, a reclining easy chair with leg extension is an option—a luxurious one, however, requiring both space and money to spare. If such is your situation, spoil yourself a little.

Chair height: Higher chairs, higher beds, higher *anything*—aid persons with hip problems and other leg conditions to stand. The lower and softer the chair, sofa, or bed is, the more *oomph* is needed to get up. Choose accordingly. If it's a beloved and often used chair that you're having trouble rising from, consider adding a firm foam cushion or temporarily putting blocks of wood under the legs. Be sure the arrangement is stable.

Sitting down and resting the injured limb on your crutches: If you are toting around a heavy cast or a painfully sprained ankle, getting it off the ground is a huge relief. When there's not an extra chair handy—and no one's suggested you slouch on their couch or bed—your crutches, all-purpose tools that they are or will come to be, will do the trick.

Soooo—first: find a place to sit. Second: place or extend a crutch directly out and under the bum leg. Third: tuck the armpit pad under the thigh of that same leg.

Presto, you now have a platform on which to heave the cast that is such a drag to drag. What's more, this maneuver—done nonchalantly and with flair—stamps you as an old hand, an expert in the crutch war, one to whom other unfortunates come for counsel and advice. So take heart; you must be getting *somewhere*—even if where you're getting doesn't seem all that exciting.

Sitting Down, Precautions

Swivel chairs, chairs on casters: These chairs are convenient and helpful, but obviously have to be used with care. Watch out particularly if you are a bit stiff or weak and likely to half fall into the chair or land off-center.

The forgetful flop: Fatigue or delirious anticipation of approaching ease sometimes leads to flopping on a bed, easy chair, or sofa *without* removing the crutches first. Picture yourself backed up, with a sophisticated angled calf touch, and flopping with the old axillaries still in place. You don't get so far, the armpits are in anguish, but—far worse—your aura of crutch capability is shattered.

Getting Down onto the Floor (Basic)

It's handy to know how you can get down onto the floor or ground to do your exercises, to play with or pick up after a small child or — if out of doors — to be ready for any and all adventures, some of which just might require locomotion on your backside. The lowdown (hah) on this maneuveur follows.

> *Note:* This requires good shoulder strength and flexibility.

Sitting: As described in "Basic Sitting Down" at the beginning of this chapter, sit yourself on the *edge* of the chair, bench, or bed. Establish your crutches nearby. The injured leg will be extended, the strong leg bent, foot flat on the floor and ready to support a good portion of your bodily mass.

> *Caution:* The knee of the uninjured leg should be without problems and with good range of motion.

Lowering to floor or ground: With your arms slightly flexed, firmly grasp the edge of the sitting surface to either side. Slide your posterior forward toward the floor or ground, removing it from its supported position on the chair edge. As you lower your body, your elbows bend increasingly. Midway in the lowering, you will quite naturally shift from supporting your upper body with your hands on the chair edge to supporting it with one elbow on the sitting surface and the opposite hand on the floor. Meanwhile your good leg is bending more and more, both at the knee and the hip as your body gradually reaches the floor.

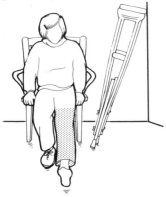 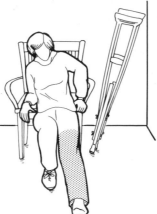 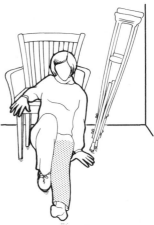

• • •Word to the Wise: FOOTSTOOL. If this maneuver is unmanage-
able, a footstool can be used as an intermediate step between chair
and floor, or bed and floor.

Getting Down onto the Floor (Advanced)

If you don't have a chair, bed, or other intermediate sitting surface,
you'll have to get down from a standing position. However, don't get
overly ambitious with such floor flopping until you are sure you are
strong and strapping. Remember—you have to get up, too.

> *Caution:* This maneuver is definitely heavy-duty, very ad-
> vanced stuff, requiring nerve and determination in addition
> to considerable strength and very good knee flexion.

Positioning: Get yourself backed up to a wall, tree, or some
other relatively flat but *extremely stable* surface. Establish your crutches
against the surface or drop them on the ground.

Lowering to the floor or ground: Pressing your back and hands
very hard against the surface, gradually move the good foot out away
from you so that you can slide your back, hands, and buttocks downward to the ground. At the very lowest level you might end up drop-
ping the final inch or two. (When you've accomplished this—and
gotten back up again, which is much harder—you'll *know* you're a sure
bet for the Crutch Hall of Fame.)

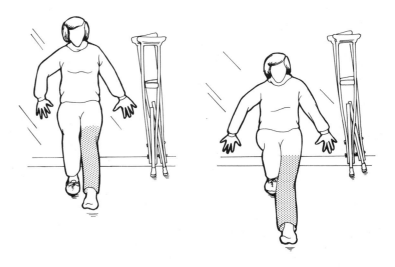

There is more physical effort involved in getting up than in getting down, but at least you don't have to aim for a target as you do when sitting. Ease of getting up is influenced by various factors including overall strength, type of injury, size of cast, and the height of the sitting surface.

Positioning: Scoot, scrunch, or inch your buttocks to the *edge* of your sitting surface so that your working foot is underneath your body. As you stand, your center of gravity will be safely established over that base of support.

Chair-touch: The calf of your good leg should be pressed against the chair—for stability when you rise and when placing the crutches under your arms.

Crutch deployment: If your uninjured leg is very strong, you can hold a crutch in each hand up near the top of its *forward* extension.

However, if that stronger leg "ain't up to snuff," pair the crutches and hold them by the *near* extension in your strong-side hand. For more detailed help for this situation see "Word-to-the-Wise" which follows.

Leg extension, push-off: Ideally, your uninjured leg does by far the majority of the work when you stand up. The crutches, grasped in each hand, are mainly for balance. So—push up, push off, straighten your knee, and you're up.

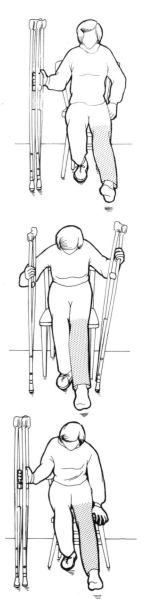

● ● ●Word to the Wise: A WEAK "STRONG" LEG. If the leg you use to get up is not strong enough for that solo performance, standing is a different story. In such a case hold the crutches together in the strong-side hand, which maximizes the lift-off push of the uninjured (but weak) leg. The hand on the injured leg side will be used where it's needed—to maximize the push-up from the seat. You will lean forward and lever yourself up with the help of the crutches on one side and the arm pushing off the sitting surface on the other side. Not quite as flashy, but the important thing is—you're up. (Some rehabilitation professionals recommend holding the paired crutches on the injured-leg side as you stand, but that loses the benefit of crutches and strong leg working together to raise body weight. It's your choice.)

Getting Up from the Floor (Basic)

Although you may think the floor is the last place you'll be when you've got a cast lashed to your leg, one never knows. If you're planning to be

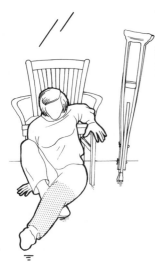

flexible and fearless and do all sorts of things despite your injury, you may *have* to get on the ground in order to manage a far-out adventure. And on the home front, any parent with a toddler to tend will appreciate the necessity of this technique.

> *Caution:* This strong-arm technique requires just that—in addition to a sturdy leg with good knee flexion.

Positioning—back: On your posterior, scoot yourself over to a chair, bench, or bed, etc., placing your back against it. Don't forget your crutches.

> *Caution:* If the object is not stationary, push it against a wall so it will be.

Positioning—elbow: With your back against the chair, place the strong-side hand onto the floor and the injured-side elbow up behind you onto the edge of the chair.

Positioning—leg: Bring your good leg up close to your buttocks, ready for maximum lift-off.

> *Caution:* Place the ankle of the injured leg on top of the uninjured leg at the ankle, so that it is not inadvertently used in any way to help raise your body.

Push off, push up: Push up *hard* with the placed hand and elbow and very hard with the good leg—in order to get your other elbow or hand onto the sitting surface. At this point you will be lying stretched out, foot on the floor, back and elbows partly on the chair, or—if the chair is low—scrunched up halfway on the chair. All depends on the height of the surface you are trying to reach.

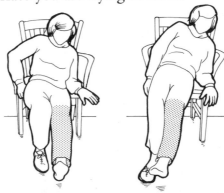

Sitting: From the double-elbow position, use your good foot to inch yourself backward and upward to help get your hands on the edge of the sitting surface. Straighten your arms, and hurrah, you should be sitting up.

Whew! It's awkward, it's ungainly, but it sure beats being helpless.

● ● ●Word to the Wise: CUSHION. If there is a sofa or chair available that is cushioned, simplify the challenge by removing the cushion so that the seat level is lowered. The lift-off requirements are agreeably reduced.

Getting Up from the Floor (Advanced)

Standing up without benefit of a helpful sitting surface is a tricky and demanding move not to be tried except when a crutch pro is desperate. But under such circumstances it's do-able, and here's how.

> *Note:* This move requires exceptional upper-body and unin-jured-leg strength, as well as knee flexibility. Men are phys-ically better equipped to do this maneuver than women.

Positioning: When no chair or similar aid is available, you will have to back yourself up to a wall, tree, or some other totally stable substitute. Draw your good foot in close to your buttocks in position for push-off.

Establishing crutches: The crutches must be placed where you can reach them for help in getting up, the tips as secure as possible to prevent them from falling.

Push off, pull up: Push up with your strong leg and the weak-side arm, while pulling up on the handgrip of the crutch leaning against the wall. Push your back tight against the surface to help lever upward. Hang in there and keep pushing up and holding on. Use anything nearby to help raise yourself, be it a boulder or branch, wall molding or ledge. This is a tough one.

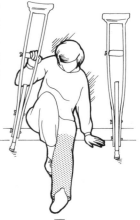

8   Simplifying Stairs

Going up or down stairs has got to be one of the most challenging tasks that the person recovering from leg injury has to face. No one who is adapting to crutches or using any mobility aid considers stairs with anything less than apprehension. It is doubtful that they will ever become what one would call fun, but there are a few tricks of the trade which will at least make flights of stairs an accepted and tolerable part of your day's routine. Do not despair, you *can* conquer stairs.

Fail-Safe Stairs, for Any and All Situations

If taking stairs in any of the advanced methods (below) is not possible due to physical trauma, lack of conditioning, or just plain terror, not to worry!—use your basic, extremely basic, way—going up or down on your backside, explained in more detail on the following pages. This may not be glamorous, but it gets you where you want to go. It's even conceivable at some future date, when you've become a famous crutch ace, that you may have to return to this most fundamental method to successfully conclude some far-out, enterprising adventure.

Lots of Stairs, with Landings

In the ABC's of crutch life (A for Apron, B for Basket, see Chapter 14) C is for Chair—and it also stands for *crucial*. C stands for chair because if you have lots of stairs to face on a frequent basis, with one or more landings, placing a chair on the landing(s) to rest on is the crutch pro's way to counteract fatigue—and thereby enhance safety. Instead of your avoiding stairs, a chair encourages freedom of movement particularly when you are weak and just learning—yet need experience in order to achieve that freedom.

Primitive as this method may seem, it is *the* fail-safe way for situations where sophisticated techniques just cannot do the job. "Pride goeth before a fall," it's said. In this case, you need never fall — if you'll put your pride aside. So here's to up or down — using the most basic method of all.

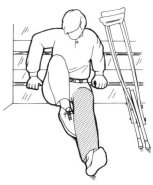

    The "bottom boogie":   Using a wall, the banister, or anything handy as support, lower yourself down onto the lowest or highest step and hitch your way — on your bottom — up or down in the desired direction. To go up, your back is to the stairs, and you place your hands behind you on the step just above. Raise your body to the same step. To come down, your feet go first, with your arms lowering your body. Don't forget your crutches. For help with getting down to the floor in the first place, see Chapter 7.

    Bottoms up: Getting up and standing again on your good foot may be a bit difficult. Use the banister or whatever is available to help raise yourself, while pushing up hard with your healthy leg.

Basic Ascending for the Non-Weight-Bearing

Going up stairs is definitely easier than coming down, but it still can be a formidable undertaking, particularly if you're recovering from surgery or if upper-body workouts have not been tops on your schedule in recent years. The following technique assumes you're using crutches and are in weakened physical condition, and recommends partial support of the body by placement of the forearm on the banister. The forearm helps in the task of ascending rather than placing total reliance on arm and shoulder strength. In addition to the physical advantage is the mental one: leaning on a friendly banister when one is starting out makes all the difference. So — do *not* fret, do *not* panic — and here goes.

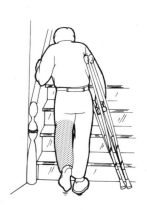

    Crutch tuck: Facing the bottom stair, tuck *both* crutches firmly under the armpit on the side farthest away from the banister.

    Facing front: Be sure the crutches are facing front, so those protruding nuts do not trip you up. The crutches will be angled about six inches to the side.

    Injured leg: Placement of the injured limb is in a flexed position next to the good leg or slightly behind, to avoid catching the cast or toes.

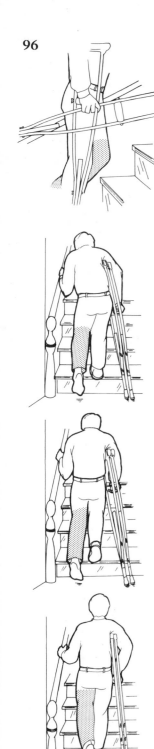

Note: If your hands are small, one crutch is turned on its side and, at the place where it balances properly, is grasped by its wooden extension simultaneously with the handgrips of the crutch you are using.

Banister support: Hold on to the banister with the hand nearest to it, placing your full *forearm* in contact and *leaning* on it for support. Your hand hangs on (this is how you get the confidence to try stairs) and pulls up; the lower arm is your support, and the upper arm does virtually nothing—simply being a substitute for the other crutch.

Crutch-arm power: Your crutch arm is straight—due to the paired crutches' being angled out to the side—and it should be ready to provide your maximum push-up power. Although the position is not correct for walking with crutches, the armpit pads in this case will be pressed tight against the chest wall. All set?

Weight distribution: Suspend your weight both on the banister forearm and the crutch arm. At the same time, push up *hard* with the crutch arm.

At this point your weight will be, momentarily, supported entirely on the paired crutches and the banister—and you will easily be able to step up your healthy foot.

Step up: So, do it. Bend up your good knee, place your foot onto the step, then use your good leg muscles to push up and straighten it. Your weight has now been transferred from the banister and crutches to your strong leg.

Now, believe it or not, once you've got that foot placed, you can relax. Nothing needs to be rushed with this method. Your weight is fully transferred to the leg on the stair, so you can bring the crutches up to the step when you feel like it. Catch your breath and—

Crutch placement: When ready, bring the crutches up and place them onto the stair next to your foot.

Rest, if you need to, then go onto the next stair by repeating the basic formula.

> *The basic formula for getting up stairs:*
> banister forearm support
> crutch arm push-up
> good leg step-up

At the top? Congrats. Get a crutch under each armpit, and off you go.

Intermediate Ascending for the Non-Weight-Bearing

Once you have conquered the basic, conservative method, both your muscles and confidence should be prepared to move on to the next level. The intermediate technique is similar to the basic, but requires more arm and shoulder strength.

Crutch tuck: Facing the bottom stair, place *both* crutches under the armpit on the side farthest away from the banister.

> *Note:* If your hands are small, one crutch is turned on its side and, at the place where it balances properly, is grasped by its wooden extension simultaneously with the handgrip of the crutch you are using.

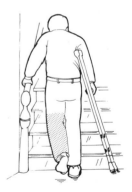

Facing front: Be sure the crutches are facing front, so those protruding nuts do not trip you up. The crutches will be angled about six inches to the side.

Injured leg: Placement of the injured limb is in a flexed position next to the good leg, to avoid catching the cast or toes.

Banister arm: Grasp the banister with the hand closest to it, keeping your arm fairly straight although with a little bend at the elbow. (Your *whole*—straightened—arm is now the substitute for the nonworking crutch held in the other hand. Your arm is *not* bent and lying on the banister.)

Crutch arm: Your crutch arm is straight—due to the paired crutches' being angled to the side—and it should be ready to provide your maximum push-up power. Although not correct for walking with crutches, the armpit pads will be pressed up against the chest wall. All set?

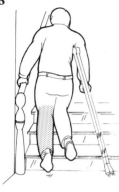

Weight distribution: Suspend your weight both on the rigid banister arm and the crutch arm. Push up *hard* with *both* arms.

At this point your weight will be momentarily supported entirely on the crutches and the banister arm—and you will easily be able to step up your healthy foot.

Step up: So, do it. Bring up your good leg, place your foot onto the step, then use your good leg muscles to push up and straighten it. Your weight has now been transferred from the banister and crutch to your strong leg.

Now, believe it or not, once you've got that foot placed, you can relax. Nothing needs to be rushed with this method. Your weight is fully transferred to the leg on the stair, so you can bring the crutches up to the stair when you feel like it. Catch your breath and—

Crutch placement: When ready, bring the crutches up and place the pair onto the stair, next to your foot. Move your banister hand up a bit into position for the next step.

Rest if you need to, then go onto the next step by repeating the formula for intermediate stair control.

> *The intermediate formula for getting up stairs:*
> banister arm and crutch arm push-up
> good leg step-up

At the top? Congrats. Get a crutch under each armpit and off you go!

Advanced Ascending for the Non-Weight-Bearing

This method is the one old-timers and pros use, a group that you will be joining before you know it. (And if the stairs you face have no banisters, the following technique is the one you'll *start* with.) It requires more strength, more balance, and more nerve, so don't try it before you're feeling pretty frisky. And remember, you can always use the fail-safe or intermediate methods when situations require it—either now or later on when ambition has taken you to fields of endeavor so challenging that cautionary tactics are called for.

● ● ●Word to the Wise: CURBS. If you are a city dweller, sidewalk curbs which are low offer good practice when you're just beginning to tackle stairs.

Caution: The first time you try a real flight of stairs by the advanced method it is wise—as well as very comforting—to have someone behind you. Your helper should stand below in the "stride" position, one foot on the stair immediately below you and his or her other foot on the stair below that. This arrangement creates the most stable position for the helper in case you totter. See Chapter 17 for more details on assistance with stairs.

Facing front: Be sure the crutches are facing front, so those protruding nuts do not trip you up.

Crutch tips: Position the tips of the crutches two or three inches from the bottom-stair lip, keeping them fairly close and on a parallel line to your body. The injured leg is held as close to one's center of gravity as possible. If it is casted, it may be slightly ahead; if uncasted, slightly behind.

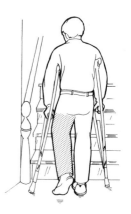

Note: Keeping the crutches in close gives you better leverage, and the distance you need to lift them is kept to a minimum.

Hand grasp: Grasp the handgrips firmly, and stiffen your arms, with the elbows slightly flexed.

Arm action: Now, straighten the arms fully and hard—so your weight is suspended completely but momentarily on your hands.

Step up: With weight distribution accomplished, bend your good leg, and step the foot up onto the stair. Depending upon your strength, that leg will straighten easily, or you will have to give an extra little "shove-up" with the arms and their crutches from their stair below.

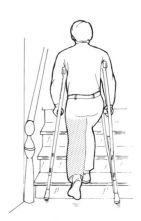

Once you've got that foot placed, you may relax and catch your breath. Take your time, and do not let anxiety make you hurry. Your crutches, on the stair below, are still steadying you. Novices think—mistakenly—that they have to rush from stair to stair, fearing their momentum will be interrupted and that they'll never make it. Not so.

Crutch arc: When ready, bring the crutches up in a slight arc and place them parallel to your foot in the middle of the stair tread. The slight arc, also used in advanced and power crutching on the flat, saves energy by reducing the distance you need to lift your body in order for the crutches to clear either the ground, floor, or stairs. This refinement is useful when stairs are climbed without pause (or panic) — in other words, when *you* are their master and not vice versa.

O.K., now it's just keep on climbing. If you get tired or anxious due to stairs that are steep or high, switch back to "intermediate." If intermediate is out because there are no banisters — and that can cause panic in itself — there is always the "bottom boogie," the fail-safe method for every situation.

Remember, at no time do you need to rush this procedure. Once again, here is the "fabulous formula" for advanced stair control.

The advanced formula for getting up stairs:
get ready
straighten your arms and suspend weight
place the strong foot on the next stair
relax and bring crutches up when ready

As you get stronger, you'll be swinging the crutches up at the same time you push off and place the foot. By then stairs will be — if not beloved — at least "old hat."

Descending Stairs

Looking down a flight of stairs for the first time can be intimidating to say the least, maybe even on a par with someone's first parachute jump. And like the parachutist, once you're in place, you're almost obliged to perform. Again, there's more than one way to skin a cat, so read on.

Fail-Safe Descending

Down (or up) — the most basic method of all.

Bottom boogie: Using a wall, the banister, or anything handy as support, lower yourself down onto the highest or lowest step, and hitch your way — on your bottom — up or down in the desired direction. Don't forget your crutches.

Bottoms up: Getting up and standing again on your good foot may be a bit difficult. Use the banister or whatever is available to help raise yourself, while pushing up hard with that healthy leg. See Chapter 7 for helpful tips on getting up from such a position.

If you are weak from surgery, an accident, or just plain terror—very normal—you will find this method the next safest way to go and surprisingly easy.

Facing front: Be sure the crutches are "facing front." The injured leg will generally be held in front of the body.

Crutch tuck: Take hold of the stairway banister with the hand closest to it and tuck your crutches firmly under the opposite armpit, grasping both handgrips in the same hand.

> *Note:* If your hands are small, one crutch is turned on its side and, at the place where it balances properly, is grasped by its wooden extension simultaneously with the handgrip of the crutch you are using.

Banister arm: Use the banister in place of the carried crutch, gripping the banister with the hand on that side. Keep a fairly rigid arm, but with the elbow bent. The forearm is *not* placed on the banister as in "Basic Ascending."

Toe position: Position yourself facing and close to the top stair, placing your foot so that the toes extend slightly over or beyond the stair lip. (If the toes are extended beyond the stair lip, you then have a shorter distance to the next stair, making the move both safer and more energy efficient.)

Crutch placement: Grip the banister at the same level as the step you are heading for, and place the paired crutches onto that next, lower step.

Knee bend: Now, without rushing, deeply bend that good knee and step down. The injured limb is held out in front—with the hip and/or knee flexed for better balance and to avoid catching it on the stair you've just left.

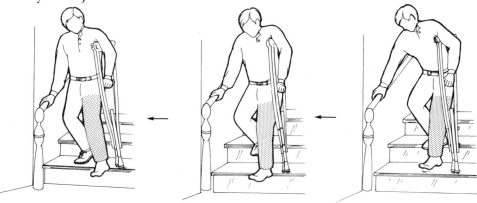

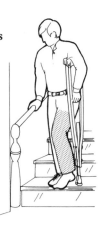

Note: The knee bend is key, for that—along with the foot placement—brings you nearer physically to the next stair, and the less distance you have to go the more confident you will feel. Since gravity is helping lower you, this basic method minimizes physical exertion, while the banister and deep knee bend maximize the feeling of stability.

Depending upon your condition and the state of your nerves, rest and regroup whenever you are firmly established on a stair. Then continue using the basic formula.

The basic formula for going down stairs:
    use the banister for support
    place your foot with the toes slightly over the edge of
        the stair
    bend the knee deeply
    step

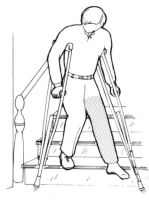

Crutch return: When—at last—you are on the bottom stair tread, support yourself by leaning against the final banister post and return one of the crutches to the other armpit. Now, place the crutches *on the floor,* bend "zee knee," and step the good foot down onto ground. Congratulations, you've arrived. That wasn't so hard, was it?

Advanced Descending for the Non-Weight-Bearing

If you've become strong, fearless, and frolicsome, this procedure will put you in the veterans' league. It's not necessarily a better way, though, being much less safe than the others, so if in doubt don't try it until after a shake-down period using the preceding, "safety-first" version. Ready? Here goes.

Facing front: As usual, be sure the crutches are "facing front." You will now have a crutch under each arm.

Toe position: Stand at the head of the stairs with the toes of the good foot slightly extending over the stair lip. Proper toe placement gives you the shortest possible distance between the stair you're on and the one you're heading for.

Crutch placement: Lean slightly and place the crutches down on the next stair, near the front of the tread and at an angle moderately away from your body and out from vertical. You are not holding on to the banister.

> *Note:* Placing the crutches near the front of the tread and on a slight slant, rather than directly vertical, lessens the distance that you have to lower your body, a refinement which is simultaneously safer and more efficient—as well as an enhancer of courage.

Knee bend: Bend your good knee *deeply,* and with your weight supported entirely on your hands for an instant, bring the bent leg forward and down, positioning the foot on the step below. Remember, so that the toes will be extending slightly over the stair lip, you will be aiming to place your *heel* between the crutch tips.

Leg straightening: As the good leg comes forward, try to straighten it in the instant before the foot is placed onto the stair, so your body does not need to be lowered farther than necessary. This is a subtle refinement that will come with experience and practice.

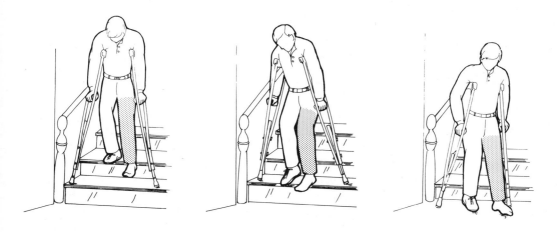

● ● ●Word to the Wise: GAP. When poised at the top of a steep set of stairs, you'll appreciate the wisdom of keeping that gap—the distance you must lower yourself—as small as possible.

With both the good foot and your crutches on that lower stair, you've conquered the first of many. You can regroup now and then continue, remembering that to impress the cheering crowds the key points are as follows:

> *The advanced formula for descending stairs:*
> > toes placed beyond the stair lip
> > crutches placed at an angle at the front of the lower stair tread
> > knee deeply bent
> > straightening of the leg

Now at last you've really got stair control. "A piece of cake!"

Additional Tips for Stairs That Are Especially Steep

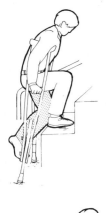

You are sometimes faced with especially steep stairs that have extra-high risers, possibly in a home but frequently encountered in trucks, recreational vehicles, or the like. Think back to advanced stair-climbing technique, where you were advised that you didn't have to rush to bring your crutches up to the stair at the same time that you planted your foot.

Advanced stair-climbing formula: Here it is again—the magic formula. Facing and properly positioned at the bottom of the stair, use maximum arm power to push off *extra* hard with your crutches, propelling your foot up and over that mountainous riser. Leave those crutches planted behind you till you're well established. Since the good foot will be up on a higher-than-normal stair, the corresponding knee will be in a *very, very* flexed position at this stage, and your weight will be suspended behind you on the planted crutches. (Therapy professionals discourage such antics for anyone in less than optimum shape.) Nothing outrageous here for the crutch pro, however, although there *is* a bit of drama, and you *do* need to be strong.

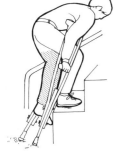

Push off, leg thrust: You'll then have to vigorously, *very* vigorously, push off with the crutches to bring them up to that towering stair while forcefully, *very* forcefully, straightening the good leg.

At this point, you can definitely, *very* definitely, take a bow.

"Stars on Stairs": Carrying Things, Up or Down

This is not an insuperable problem even if one does not have a spouse, cooperative offspring, or some other full-time, able-bodied live-in available. Transportation in general is dealt with in Chapter 14, but for now let's just point out the obvious.

The drop: A plentiful variety of objects can get downstairs just by being dropped in the proper direction.

The heave: Ditto for upstairs, only the operative verb is "thrown" or "tossed." Normally, the process of chucking articles *up* the stairs has to be repeated several times, necessitating some advanced crutch technique, but—if you want to get the object up there bad enough, you can and probably will do it. For more details, see Chapter 14.

Caution: Picking up objects in the middle of a flight of stairs is advanced technique requiring good balance and crutch skills.

Ascending or Descending Stairs: Partial-Weight-Bearing

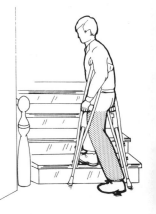

Compared to the challenges that stairs present for non-weight-bearers, having two legs to share the work is considered heaven. Balance is decidedly less of a concern, and physical strength not as important. Nevertheless, one or both of those lower legs may be weak or injured —so it "ain't necessarily so" that taking stairs is a field day for the partial-weight-bearing. Determination to recover strength and function, to enlarge your range of activities—and perseverance in doing so—will still be required.

Ascending for the Partial-Weight-Bearing Formula: The good leg (foot) always steps up first. That leg which is stronger is asked to do the job. In the case of *climbing* stairs, more strength is required to step up onto the next step—to raise your body weight and to straighten the leg afterward. So the stronger leg steps first.

Descending for the Partial-Weight-Bearing Formula: The injured leg (foot) always steps down first. Stepping down requires the least effort—so the weak leg starts off. Considerable flexibility and range of motion are needed for the leg that *follows,* which has to bend deeply. It also has to be strong enough to hold your body weight while the weaker one steps down. So, the good leg follows after the weaker leg goes first.

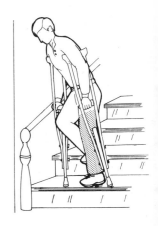

One therapist helps his patients remember this way, although it seems unnecessary: "The good go to heaven; the bad go to hell." The good leg goes first when going *up*—to heaven. The bad leg goes first when going *down,* to hell. Don't let those suggestions scare you—go anywhere you please.

> *Caution:* An escalator is such a tricky proposition for a person on crutches that attempting one is not recommended for anyone who is non-weight-bearing, especially if he is on his own. Even with aid, the non-weight-bearing individual would be well advised to seek some other means of ascent or descent. A building possessing an escalator will have elevators or stairs available as well.

Approach: Approach the beginning of the escalator closely, and place both crutches under the *weak-side* armpit.

Railing clutch: Be prepared to grab on to the moving railing with the strong-side hand.

Step on, good leg: Step onto the moving stair with your good foot, holding on to the railing with the hand on the same side.

Step on, bad leg: Bring the weaker leg and the crutches onto the stair. Your weight will be partially supported by them as the escalator rises or descends.

Escape: At the end be prepared to step off with your strong leg, which means—since the crutches will be useless on the moving stair when it arrives at the bottom or top—that for an instant your weight will be on the weak leg.

> *Caution:* You will not be able to do ride escalators *unless* your injured leg is *truly* partially-weight-bearing. Nor is it advisable to try this escapade alone the first time, unless you are really a "supercrutch."

Elevators

The main challenge of elevators is getting in and out without the doors' doing anything nasty. Chapter 9 deals with doors in general. There you will find related techniques—such as wedging—explained in conjunction with "heavy-duty doors," and dealing with crowds discussed in conjunction with revolving doors.

As in crossing streets or other situations where there are likely to be crowds, take your time to assess the "traffic patterns." Ask someone to follow you into the elevator and fend people off if the press of a crowd might be hard enough to knock you over.

• • •Word to the Wise: HOLD BUTTON. Needless to say, your greatest protection against the doors closing on you is the door-hold button. Someone will be glad to press it for you as you enter, and if you're a bit shaky, be sure to press it yourself before exiting.

Precautions on Stairs

Handrails: Handrails, if not present, should be installed on both sides of hazardous stairs if necessary. They are best extended beyond the top and lowest step, because support is needed when getting on and off those steps.

Aid: In some situations it is advisable to have someone behind you simply for safety's sake. In other situations — for instance, on extremely steep stairs or ramps such as those associated with docks at low tide — a person behind pushing at the buttocks level can make the crucial difference between going up in the extremely basic fail-safe mode or the advanced mode.

Safety belt: In conjunction with aid from a friend or family member, a commercially available safety (or "gait") belt can be worn by the individual who is too weak, overweight, or fearful when climbing stairs. Holding on to clothing or a regular belt may be risky unless the material is unquestionably sturdy enough. See Chapter 17 for details on how you can help correctly and safely.

Lighting: Be sure it is uniform and there are no dark areas. A night light, a spot light like those used to dramatize pictures (floor model), or even Gro-Lights for plants — can temporarily be focused on stairs.

Open stair risers: If the spaces between the stair treads have nothing filling them in, they can be a serious tripping hazard. Be extra cautious that the stepping (good) foot does not get placed too far forward and that the toes of the bad leg do not get caught underneath the stair ledge. If necessary, at least in your own home, open risers can easily be closed with planks of wood.

9 Doors Made Passable

Doors rate a chapter all to themselves, due to the very real difficulties they can present to the uninitiated person using crutches or other mobility aids. Not to worry—read on for freedom from fear. The techniques you learn here will enable you to vanquish any portal—from your own front door to the heavy-weights of commercial buildings, some of which are capable of stopping Superman in his tracks.

● ● ●Word to the Wise: DISTANCE. The most basic requirement for the opening of any door is judging the distance you need to be from the door in question in order to open it without your body getting in the way. Generally speaking, the distance you need to be from the door relates to its width—but other factors are its weight, your strength, and your crutch skills. Experience will be the best teacher, but normally you'll want to *overestimate* the distance. It is easier to move forward to the door in adjusting distance than to hop backward—and that saves energy.

In general, safety is maximized if you avoid lunging and over-using body leverage—which can upset your balance.

If a door is impassable due to whatever reason (type of injury, weakness, door too narrow for wheelchair passage) and its location permits, consider temporarily leaving it open, removing it, propping it, or tying it back. In the case of two doors, such as a screen and door combo, expenditure of energy—as well as time and frustration—will be immeasurably reduced by simplification in some form or other.

Simple, Plain, Everyday Doors

When you have judged the proper distance, the technique for opening simple doors is as follows:

Stabilization: Be well stablized on your crutches.

Armpit grip: Have the strong-side crutch held in the armpit grip to free your hand for grasping the door handle. See Chapters 5 and 14 for more on the armpit grip.

Door pull: Then—having stationed yourself the proper distance from the door, lean forward to get the handle and pull the door toward you. To save energy, only open the door wide enough to pass through.

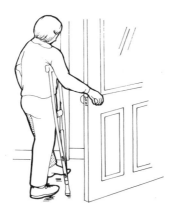

> ***Note:*** The weight of the door is a major consideration, and again—with practice—you'll be adjusting to how much heft and haul you require for each type.

Door close: At this point, with a simple door, the job is finished. Go on through, but don't get too carried away; stay within reach so that you can turn and close the door behind you.

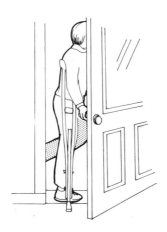

Simple Doors with Pneumatic Closing Devices

This type of door does not present a problem if you attack it logically, which means setting the small locking tab of the pneumatic device in place so the door will stay open while you pass through. This holds true whether you need to pull the door open toward you first and then set the locking device, or push the door away from you before setting it. In either case here's how to go about it.

Free hand: Free up a hand by leaning your off-side crutch against the door frame, the wall, or your own waist. For more on establishing crutches against your own body see "Picking Up Objects" in Chapter 14.

Crutch wedge: Approach the door and pull it toward you or push it open away from you as required, using the near-side crutch as a wedge—or door stop—against the bottom to keep it ajar.

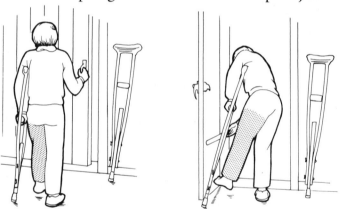

Set tab: Depending on the location of the pneumatic device, lean down or reach up to set the locking tab by sliding it against the pneumatic tube and wedging it there.

Walk on through: O.K., you've now got the door subdued, so just grab the crutch you put aside and pass on through.

Tab release: Use the same process to release the locking tab. The door will slowly close on its own, and you're on your way. Not too terrible, was it?

Caution: Be sure that the locking tab on such a door actually does its job before trusting your already impaired self to its operation. If *it* is impaired too, treat the door as a heavy-duty type, see below.

Simple doors placed at the top of stairs do not usually present problems any different from those presented by doors in general, although you naturally proceed extra cautiously because — after all — you are perched (like Humpty Dumpty) at the top of a fall.

Doors with Pneumatic Devices in Combination with Stairs

Such doors are a different matter, however. If you are on stairs on the outside or down side of such a door, you are required to pull it open toward you before wedging the locking tab, and the lack of room on the stair definitely makes such a maneuver become an advanced technique. If you are very confident and very experienced, as well as determined, the experts attack this way:

Positioning: At a suitable distance from the door, stand well over to the side of the stair.

Crutch wedge: Pull open the door and quickly wedge a crutch and your body into the opening, pushing the door open wide at the same time. You'll have to be hanging tough here.

Set tab: Set the locking tab, just as you would do for simple doors with pneumatic closing devices. Enter or pass through. Whew! *Not* a trick for the faint of heart.

> *Caution:* Such doors can be mastered, but do not try them unless you are an old hand at this game — and are seeking challenges. This is a time when total independence is not advised, so get help if any is available. If no one is around remove the pneumatic closure if this will be a frequent problem or use that method of last resort, which is to sit down and handle stair, door, and pneumatic closure on your backside. Since even that may not always be possible, the worst-case scenario is that you may have to find another way in.

Heavy-Duty Doors

These are the large, sometimes extremely heavy doors that you encounter in commercial buildings and public places such as post offices, airports, banks, rest rooms, stores, museums, and the like. There's not much chance of avoiding them, because their function is control of security, energy, noise, and fire — matters of increasing concern in public places. The technique for coping with big doors is definitely advanced, but you need to master doors such as these in order to be the independent entrepreneur you want to be. "Attack" is the operative word, since strength — as well as some quick and slick moves — is required to dominate the situation.

● ● ●Word to the Wise: ADJUSTMENT. A little-known fact is that many such doors can be adjusted to vary the amount of effort needed to open them. There are regulations governing the allowable pressure: five pounds — applied at the handle — for interior doors and eight pounds for exterior. If you are subjected to an unequal struggle with doors of this type, consider asking that there be a readjustment. A lighter door is safer, much easier to wedge, and saves energy. Read on for battle plans designed for varying types of these monsters, and how to outflank them.

Heavy Doors that Open Toward You

Positioning: Station yourself the correct distance away from the door, being sure you are well balanced.

Door haul: Take a deep breath, flex those muscles, and using the armpit grip to free up a hand, *haul* that door toward you. For more on the armpit grip, see Chapters 5 and 14.

You may wish your biceps were brawnier, but stay with it. As your experience increases, that "heave 'n' haul" will seem less of an effort, but at this stage you'll probably have to put a lot of *oomph* into it. Once you've got the door back, success is beckoning, but some tricky two-steps remain to be danced before you can celebrate. That door is open, but you have to get through without the monster knocking you over or nipping your heels.

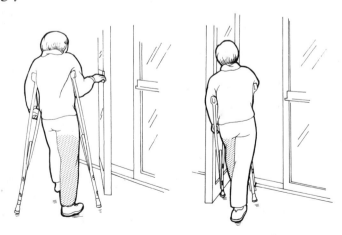

Crutch wedge: Give the door another sharp tug toward you, let go, and quickly place the near crutch tip right at the bottom of the door, jamming it there and wedging the door open. An optional way of wedging it open is to tug hard, then let go and take a quick hop and pivot combined — so that your hip or back is against the door, holding it ajar. This is not as efficient, but may be easier to start with.

The hop: Either way, you will have taken a hop forward while wedging the crutch tip or using your back as the wedge.

Wedging, repulsing: To continue going through, you will need to remove the wedged tip and rewedge it farther ahead, accompanied by another forward hop and perhaps an elbow-hip repulse or two.

A couple of these tricky steps should pretty well finish off the door, with your final fling being another firm repulse as you depart — to keep it from counterattacking when your back is turned.

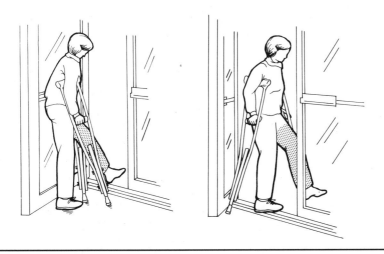

Note: Sometimes the crutch tip gets trapped between the bottom of the door and the floor — due to your excellent wedging prowess. No need to panic. Use the armpit grip to free up a hand, push the door slightly away from you to release the trapped tip, then resume the battle.

Heavy Doors that Push Open

Hip strike: Get pretty close to the door, then partially pivot so that your hip is in a position to push. Be sure your balance is good, then commence your hip action — pushing the door outward away from you.

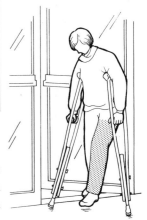

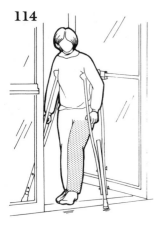

Wedging: As the door opens, follow the bottom edge using your crutch as a door stop, wedging it and hopping sideways along the door until you are through. Another way is to sustain the action you started with—continue to push it open with your hip and back while making your way through. Be on the alert that your foe doesn't give you a parting blow as you leave the field of battle.

Advanced Procedures to Push Open Heavy Doors

Double-handed shove: This is an all-out attack, encompassing a close approach to the door and then—both crutches held in the armpit grip—a determined, vigorous shove with both hands to thrust it away from you.

Wedging: As the door opens, quickly replace the crutch under the other armpit, take a hop forward, and wedge your near-side crutch at the bottom of the door to keep it from shutting. Hop and wedge alternately until the door is finished off.

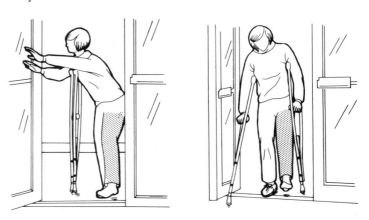

In the beginning you may want to use your shoulder or back to help fend off the weight of the door, when either your strength or your balance is not yet fully tuned up. And on the other hand, a super-advanced crutchjock can attack such a door with a shove strong enough to allow passing through with only one wedging, or maybe none at all. (At that stage it is promised that crutch connoisseurs will not be mistaking you for a mere dabbling amateur.)

The view ahead: If the door that you are attempting to open is solid and you cannot see through it, be on the alert for some other person opening it from the far side. Your equilibrium is dependent upon your wedged crutch and body weight counterbalancing the weight of the door, and this balance is alarmingly upset when the door is unexpectedly pulled on by someone else. This scenario is not as rare as it might seem and provides a scare for all involved. *Watch out.*

"*Help*" *from behind:*   Less obvious, but providing the same sort of unsettling surprise, is the person who comes up behind you and helpfully gives the door a shove just when most of your strength and weight are concentrated against it in the effort of opening. Needless to say, the passerby is attempting to be of aid, so try to be gracious as you flail around regaining your balance— but once again, watch out.

Elevator Doors

The trick here, of course, is to get in or out safely, but unless the elevator is particularly speedy off the mark, or there is a large and pushy crowd that refuses to either let you in first or to hold open the door for you, you should have little difficulty. Just remember the following points:

Be ready: Be physically prepared, and enter or leave quickly once the doors open. There's really plenty of time, but err on the side of caution. If the doors are closing, let them go—don't try and jump through. When people are really pushy and piggy, enlist a passerby——first, to protect you from behind, and second, to pry a place for you once inside.

Stability: If the elevator rises very fast or is unstable for some other reason, hold on to the safety rail or establish yourself up against the back or side of the car.

Door-hold button: If you are uncertain about getting through speedy elevator doors, the really safe way to enter is to push the safety button that holds the door open. Since the button is inside the elevator, help from a passerby is recommended at this point.

Leave-taking: To exit, move out fast or employ the door-hold safety button, particularly if there is a crowd.

Precautions, Urban Settings

Elevator banks: In city office buildings and department stores there are generally "banks" of grouped elevators. Be restrained—pick one elevator and stay there until it comes rather than rushing to another one that arrives first.

Crowds: The urban scene can frequently place you in the midst of busy, often thoughtless people who in getting themselves on elevators or escalators or performing other tasks prevent you from performing yours. Here you must ask for help, both to accomplish your mission and for your own safety.

Subways: Managing entry into a subway car at peak periods is hazardous and should be avoided if possible. If impossible, ride the subway in the company of an associate or friend or ask someone to help you get on and get off. The latter solution is not without risk, but neither is the subway. If at all feasible, when making your way to the platform have your companion follow just behind you to keep faster-moving people from mowing you down.

Revolving Doors

The wrinkle of revolving doors lies in the fact that you do not have control over entry into the apparatus or the door's speed. This means unfortunately that unless absolutely no one is around—unlikely with doors such as these, which are generally located in busy areas—you will have to depend upon some public-spirited being to follow you in the next slot to keep the door from being revolved too fast for your rate of progress. Such souls do exist, however, so no need to hold back. Equally advisable is that when you enter the apparatus there should be no people ahead of you to drag you along in their wake.

Although modern safety precautions may require that such doors be locked, there is usually a conventional door nearby that may be safer than the revolving door.

Bathroom: Starting Your Day Right 10

Bathroom procedures present real challenges for persons recovering from any type of leg injury or surgery. Besides sensible concern for safety, there's plain exasperation with the increased time it takes to accomplish necessary health, cleanliness, or beauty routines. Stay tuned: the following suggestions will help you get to work or wherever you're going safely and — if you pay proper attention — without having to get up more than 15 minutes earlier than you used to.

• • •Word to the Wise: CHAIR. C is for Chair, part of the ABC triad of Absolutely Basic Cargo for persons gimping and limping along. See Chapter 14 for A — apron, and B — basket. In addition to the crucial "chair for stairs" recommended in Chapter 8, there is also a crucial chair for the bathroom — sturdy, straight-backed, and light enough for you to move by yourself. Or if you have good stability, it can be a swiveling office-type chair on casters. To protect the chair from dampness and to prevent slipping, place a folded terry towel on the seat.

Sponge Baths and Sink Shampoos

Caution: Avoid showers at first. If you are weak after surgery or extended bed rest, do not undertake showering until you have regained strength and balance. The process of showering when non-weight-bearing or lugging a cast is complicated, time-consuming, and very fatiguing. Involved are not only the lengthy processes of bathing but those of organizing clothing, drying, and dressing as well.

However, daily bathing is important for other things besides cleansing and enhanced blood circulation in the skin. A presentable "exterior you" generally means a happier "interior you." The answer for this situation is sponge baths and sink shampoos.

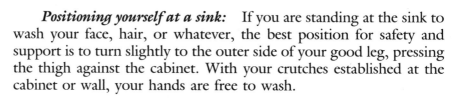

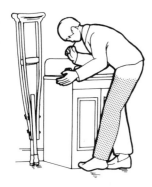

Chair positioning: Ideally, placement should be within reaching distance of the sink so you can collapse onto the chair between health or beauty-related chores such as shaving, applying makeup, or styling hair.

● ● ●Word to the Wise: TOILET. If there is not enough room in your bathroom for a chair as described, the toilet seat will become the logical place for some of those chores. If sitting is difficult because of the low height of the toilet seat, temporary seat raisers are available from your local medical-supply store. Walker-type railings are also helpful. Portable, wrap-around railings are available that do not need installation. See Chapter 19 for how to obtain these aids by mail order.

Positioning yourself at a sink: If you are standing at the sink to wash your face, hair, or whatever, the best position for safety and support is to turn slightly to the outer side of your good leg, pressing the thigh against the cabinet. With your crutches established at the cabinet or wall, your hands are free to wash.

● ● ●Word to the Wise: POSITION. The usual position of facing the sink cabinet results in an awkward stance with both your bent knees fighting the cabinet, very poor stability, and inability to use your hands freely and fully.

Sink shampoos: Freshly washed hair is a morale-booster—as well as a necessity—but the catch is that showering in order to have clean hair consumes a lot of time and energy. The solution, of course, is to shampoo in the sink when you are in a hurry or if overall bathing is not required. Dry shampoo is another possibility.

● ● ●Word to the Wise: KITCHEN. If your bathroom sink is small or low—use the kitchen sink. The increased height is a big help, and better yet, kitchen sinks often have flexible, dish-rinsing spray attachments which ease hair-washing immensely. Spray devices can also be purchased and attached to existing sink or tub faucets.

Sponge bathing: Generally—if privacy can be maintained— sponge bathing is also easier in the kitchen. The height of the sink is perfect for a person in any stage of recovery, there is generally more "elbow room," the taller cabinet improves balance, and kitchen floors are made to be washed so spills are not a problem.

Assistance: A prudent approach is not to be alone on your first attempt at taking a shower or bath. At the very least, have someone within calling distance in case you unexpectedly need help.

Mat: A rubber nonslip mat *must* be on the tub or shower-stall floor. Most bathroom accidents are caused by a slippery tub or shower bottom. Additionally, beware of bathtub bottoms that are curved rather than squared-off and flat.

Damp floors: Be especially careful of damp floors. Beach-type slippers with rubber soles are safer than bare feet.

Rugs: Scatter rugs are as hazardous in the bathroom as anywhere else, despite the fact that they counteract slippery tiles. Remove them or fasten them down securely with double-faced rug tape.

Chair: Remember—if you have a castered chair, it is not stable for leaning on. To keep a regular chair from sliding, rubber leg-tips can be added, or it can be placed on a nonslip rubber mat.

Bathing with cast, bandage, or brace: In general, you will not want to get these wet. There are latex protectors available which offer much better protection—and correspondingly more enjoyable bathing—than plastic garbage bags. Check at your pharmacy or medical-supply store, or see Chapter 19.

Cast protectors: Latex protectors, when wet, are very slippery and can be a hazard in themselves. Be sure you stabilize yourself properly—and take it slow.

Glass bottles and bars of soap: Avoid using these in the shower. Shampoos and rinses should be in plastic bottles or tubes. Soap is best in pump dispensers or on soap ropes.

Grab bars: For recoveries of long duration, grab bars for getting in and out make your tub or shower infinitely more accessible and safer. Available at medical-supply stores or hardware stores, they can be self-installed if carefully aligned with underlying wall supports. See Chapter 19 for mail-order options.

Caution: Do not support yourself on objects not made for that function, such as wall-mounted soap dishes, towel racks, etc.

Entering Showers and Bathtubs

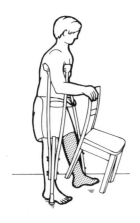

Positioning: The first step in getting ready to bathe is to position the all-important bathroom chair directly up against the bathtub or shower stall. The chair should be positioned in the direction that places the *good leg* on the side closest to the tub.

> *Note:* You may have to move your chair from its regular position near the sink or wherever you use it in daily dressing or bathroom routines. Although the maneuver is a bit advanced, there is no need to send up an S.O.S., you can move the chair yourself. Here's how. With your crutches stable and under each arm as usual, use your armpit-grip and strong-side hand combo to pick up the chair and place it in front of you. Crutch yourself forward to the chair, then pick up and move it ahead again. Little shove by little heave will get it to the desired spot. If the chair is castered, just use the "armpit-grip push." See Chapter 14 for an explanation of the extremely useful "armpit-grip carry."

Organization: Be sure your soap, shampoo, razor, shaving cream, etc., are in the bath or shower enclosure and that another towel for drying off (besides the one on the chair seat) is available on the back of the chair. Turn on the shower water—either from a seated position on your chair or standing if you can manage it safely.

Swing over: Sitting with your *good leg* closest to the tub or shower stall, swing it over the side of the tub or into the stall. Place your foot onto the nonskid mat, grasp either the sides of the stall, bath enclosure, grab bars, or doors, and pull yourself up.

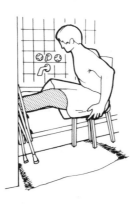
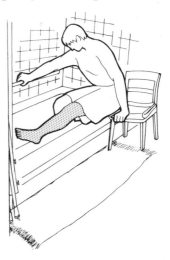

> *Caution:* Any supports must be absolutely sturdy and stable.

Hang on: If you are not using a tub or shower seat—(when out of your own quarters it's unlikely there will be one)—hold on to or balance against anything at hand that is *stable*. This may be sliding tub doors, stall frame, grab bars if they exist, shower-curtain rod or, lacking anything else, bracing one hand against the wall while washing with the other. Needless to say, in all such adventuresome situations prudence and caution are paramount. (See below for thoughts on tub and shower seats.)

Wash and rinse: At this point you wet, wash, and rinse yourself while balancing on your good leg, hopping around as required to be properly situated in the stream of shower water and holding on with whatever hand is not being used.

> *Caution:* Standing and bathing in a tub or shower stall while managing a leg injury requires good judgment in addition to advanced crutch skills, strength, and balance.

If you have no tub or shower chair, return to your bathroom chair to rest when needed. (The technique for exiting the bath or shower is explained below.) To save energy while you are sitting (and wet), do any required shaving at this time.

Bathing Accessories

Transfer bench, shower chair, tub seat: Helpmates for bathing— such as water-resistant transfer benches, shower chairs, or tub seats— are available from medical-supply stores or through mail order (see Chapter 19). A transfer bench is one which extends from outside the tub to inside the tub, with rubber-tipped legs at each end. It is the easiest and safest method for getting in, particularly with a heavy cast. Because of the vastly improved safety it affords, as well as comfort in bathing, such a seat or bench is highly recommended, particularly if you are a bit shaky or are going to be non-weight-bearing for quite awhile.

Although such equipment does not permit luxuriating in the water itself, seats and benches do allow a relaxed, safe, and thorough wash-up. (Any expendable chair or stool can be used if you have one, as long as it is centered on a rubber mat.) If you are in a cast and there's space enough, position your crutch under your thigh, as described in Chapter 5. Place the other end on the tub ledge, and put the cast on top to keep it dry.

Note: Taking a "real" bath, by the way, is almost impossible for the non-weight-bearing individual because of the difficulty in getting up from the bottom of a bathtub. If help is available, however, you may be able to manage. Suffice it to say that if such a person is so advanced as to be able to self-elevate from the bottom of a tub, he or she need read no further.

Spray hose: If you use a seat of some sort, an extremely helpful item is a flexible spray hose attached to the faucet—or temporarily replacing the existing shower head—so that you can sit and wash yourself all over while conserving energy. These flexible hoses are also very useful for shampooing at bathroom or kitchen sinks and are available at medical-supply houses, hardware and houseware stores, and through mail order.

Leaving Showers or Bathtubs

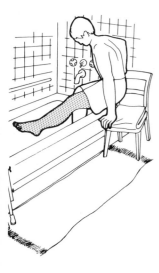

Positioning: Stabilize yourself, and hop to the exit side of the tub or stall, positioning your injured *limb* as close as possible to the edge.

Pivot and sit: Pivot slightly on your good foot, so that your backside is facing the chair placed just outside the tub. Carefully "poke your posterior" across the tub side or shower-stall ledge to a position on the towel-covered chair.

At this stage, both legs will still be in the tub. Drying off can be done either now—before you have removed your legs—or after.

• • •Word to the Wise: DRYING. When coping with a leg injury of any kind, it is always safer to dry off when sitting down.

Remove legs: If you haven't already removed your legs from inside the tub, carefully maneuver the injured leg out first, then the other leg.

Now—relax. You're probably pretty worn out, but it was worth it: you are fresh and clean.

Sitting down on a toilet or getting up is similar to techniques covered in Chapter 7. For brief review, see below.

Positioning: Approach the toilet and turn around, positioned so that the side of the good-leg calf is pressed against the toilet seat and bowl—with the leg rather straight and rigid.

The stability of that position allows you to get pants lowered or skirts hitched up without teetering or tottering—the last thing you need at this crucial (and sometimes rushed) stage.

Sitting: Sit down with the help of your crutches in one hand and by putting the other hand down onto the seat to slow your descent.

Caution: Toilet-seat heights are variable and often are lower than chair heights you are accustomed to. Be cautious and careful. The reason, according to reliable rumor, that toilet seats are low is because of the anatomical design of the human body. It seems the elimination system is better stimulated if knees are slightly above the level of hips. A low toilet seat accomplishes this laudable goal; however, it sure makes the other goal—of sitting down and getting up—harder for persons with arthritis or recovering from leg injury.

• • •Word to the Wise: ARMRESTS, SEAT. If you are weak, have problems with balance, find the weight of a cast difficult to manage, or are perennially overrushed in making it to the toilet, adjustable arm rests are available that wrap around the toilet and are used as railings. Similar in looks to walkers, and sometimes combined with a walker, they can be obtained at medical-supply stores and need no installation. Another device that may be helpful is an add-on toilet seat that raises the existing seat's height. This is particularly helpful after hip surgery or any situation of diminished physical strength. See Chapter 19 for obtaining the toilet safety rail or seat through mail order.

"Production Problems"

When your normal exercise patterns and daily routines are severely curtailed or interrupted, bowel movements can become difficult, painful, time-consuming, and sometimes almost impossible.

Stool softeners: One solution is a stool softener, a nonprescription product, that helps to produce a soft stool that passes regularly, painlessly, and without urgency. Not a laxative, it can be used without risk of your becoming dependent on it; permanent or long-term use, however, is to be avoided. Do not be alarmed if bowel normalcy is slow in returning even after resumption of walking and usual exercise; time and the return to your regular lifestyle will allow you to taper off softeners and eliminate them entirely.

Check with your doctor before using these, and make sure the stool softener is that only, not a combination softener and laxative, which can be habit-forming.

● ● ●Word to the Wise: MEALS. When digestion and plumbing are sluggish, eat more frequently and avoid big meals.

"Morning Rush – The Moment of Truth"

Some people, slowed down by their injury or crutches — or both — have problems getting to the toilet in time for urination, most frequently during or after the extended hours of nighttime rest.

Bedpan: If this annoyance persists, a bedpan, urinal, or other receptacle kept discretely at bedside may be preferable to leakage over floors or carpets. Cover it, for privacy, with a towel.

Clothing: If difficulty in getting to the toilet makes close calls a problem throughout the day, wear clothing that can easily be lifted up or pulled down. Elastic waists are best for pants, with stretchy suspenders to keep them in place if they are too floppy for getting around safely.

Bedroom: Getting Out on the Right Side

Leg injuries and assistive aids do not turn sleeping areas into serious threats as they do so many other areas of endeavor or activities that are taken for granted. Thankfully, bedrooms get to remain the comforting places they've always been, and that's good, because you may be spending more time there than you are used to. So—as you settle into your pillow and before you nod off, check the suggestions below. See Chapter 19 for information on all bedroom paraphernalia.

Getting into Bed

Positioning: Approach, turn around, and place yourself so that the back of your leg is touching the bed. Try to choose placement that will position your head at the pillow area when you lie down. For details on sitting and standing skills, see Chapter 7.

Hand and crutch positions: Hold the paired crutches by the handgrip on your strong-leg side. Place the other hand behind you on the mattress edge, and sit down. Establish your crutches at the head of the bed.

Levering: If the injured leg is weak or casted, you can help by placing the strong leg underneath it at the ankle level. Then use the strong leg to raise the other one.

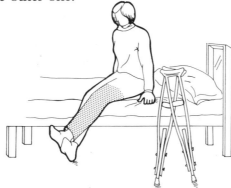

Leg swing: Hold on to the mattress edge with one hand, and have the other one behind you for support. With legs in the levering position, hoist and bring them onto the bed while rotating the buttocks and hips. Uncross your legs and lower yourself.

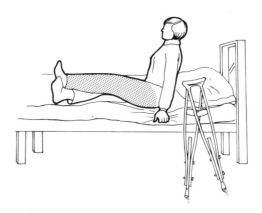

Body positioning: Use your elbows, hands, and the heel of your good leg to push yourself up into a comfortable position. Enjoy.

• • •Word to the Wise: BEDS. If you're using crutches, the large and beckoning expanse of a bed invites fast and floppy falls when mind and muscles have taken all they can bear. When flopping fast, remember to remove the crutches from under your arms *first*—or you'll be hung up in midair suspended at the armpits. (You'll avoid looking like a beginner just starting crutch kindergarten.)

Getting Out of Bed

Transport: Grab your crutches from the head of the bed and place them nearby. Your uninjured leg transports the injured leg to the side of bed as follows. Lying on your back, slide the strong foot under the casted or injured leg, move both legs to the side of the bed, and then dangle them overboard.

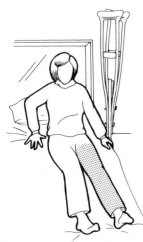

Pull-me, push-me: Pull on the mattress edge with one hand, and push up with the other hand in order to sit fully. If that is too difficult, roll onto your side toward the edge of the bed and pull and push from there—a position requiring less abdominal strength. Grab your crutches, stand, and off you go. For help with standing techniques, see Chapter 7.

Extra pillows: Extra pillows are almost always needed for elevation of an injured limb. King-size ones are best at supporting the whole leg rather than letting the foot dangle off the other end of a standard pillow. Heels that spend a lot of time in bed are prone to chafing and sores, and keeping them up on pillows can help with that, too. When you roll over onto your side, put one between your legs to prevent unpleasant pressure or cast friction. Remember, you can also get some elevation by inserting a small suitcase or books under the mattress itself. For more on elevation see Chapter 2.

Bedside water: It is hard carrying a glass of water without spilling it even if you *have* read the advanced methods of hauling explained in Chapter 14. So if you like water at odd times during the day or night, have someone place a full pitcher nearby. Later on, as a certified master of crutch techniques, you'll be able to get it there yourself.

Bedpan and urinal: Hospitals have now decreed that plastic urinals and bedpans belong to the patients. If you are hospitalized, bring yours home; you'll be glad you did. Getting to the bathroom in time after surgery of any sort can be a losing proposition, and with a leg injury or cast the odds are even worse. Place the urinal or bedpan within reach nearby—tidily tucked under a towel—if for nothing else than peace of mind. Any large-mouthed jar with a tightly fitting lid can be substituted for a urinal, and a lightweight, slim—"fracture"—bedpan can be bought for a nominal sum at a medical-supply store or through mail order.

Hospital-style, over-bed table: Good to work at and eat at, such tables can be rented at medical-supply stores.

Lazy Susan: This is such an easy trick that you may end up using it many places, and long after you've forgotten all about your knee reconstruction or broken ankle. Place a plastic lazy Susan on your bedside table or on any handy surface near where you will be spending recuperative time. On it you can place all those items which normally get increasingly far away as their numbers mount up. A television remote control, reading glasses, pen, audiocassettes, makeup, stationery, scissors, or whatever you use a lot remain accessible with a flick of the hand. Lazy Susans, small and large, are found at most hardware or home-furnishing stores. Use them wherever improved accessibility—such as in kitchen cabinets or the refrigerator—is needed.

Over-lap bed tray: These trays straddle your legs on legs of their own, and frequently have storage compartments on each side for magazines, newspapers, and other items. They can be found in mail-order catalogues and department stores.

Beanbag-type lap table or desk: This is another type of working surface designed for the person sitting down, either in bed or elsewhere. It is portable and does a wonderful job conforming to your lap and not slipping off. Great for meals, correspondence, and business — including your laptop computer — wherever you have settled yourself. Available at department stores and mail-order outlets.

Mattress pocket: A storage pocket, one end of which is tucked between the spring and mattress, is handy on the side of a bed or sofa to hold reading glasses, writing materials, and other frequently used items. Get a friend to make one, use the lower half of a pocketed apron (tuck in the bib part), or check department stores, bedding stores, and catalogues.

Baskets: Lightweight plastic baskets of all sizes are found at hardware or home-furnishing stores, and are pefect for your bedside table, the bed itself, or your designated dressing area. Organize your toiletries and grooming supplies for easy use and saving of precious time. If you need office or desk materials, they can be centralized in the same fashion. You'll find with any type of walking impairment that such baskets are easily transportable so that you can vary your locale safely and with minimum use of energy.

Remote-control TV: Laid up as you are, think how a remote-control apparatus would simplify your television viewing. More important, remote control saves a great deal of energy and dampens the frustration factor enormously. (Is that excuse enough? Trade your extinct model in or rent a remote-control TV temporarily.)

Night clothes: Strange advice as it may seem, slinky garments make it easier to move around in bed because they slide rather than clutch. Casts, general weakness, and post-op fatigue make such efforts energy-depleting and annoying. Satin sheets would ease things even more, but unless you have a fairy godmother, just try to wear night clothes that glide rather than grip.

Night lights: Safety requires that you don't risk a fall when you are hampered by a stiff and painful leg injury or are using crutches, cane, or walker. Have a night light in your bedroom and bathroom, as well as the hallway and stairs if you'll be using them after dark.

Making the Bed

If a tidy bed is a joy forever in your life yet there are no slaves around to tidy it for you, do not feel you have to settle for the sin of slothfulness.

Be creative, and you will discover that you can do a good deal of the making before you even get out of bed. (The whole subject depends on whether your pleasure is a neat nest or a rumpled roost.) Fast—but not hard—rules follow:

Sit: Fold up extra blankets or quilts and lay them aside or at the foot of the bed. Pull up, straighten, and smooth out the top sheet and blankets as best you can. Plump up and organize your pillows as best you can.

Exit: Disarrange your top layer as little as possible in getting out. Your departure must be of a sliding, slithery sort so as not to undo your just-made bed.

Balance: In order to do a little more organizing, balance yourself by pressing the uninjured leg and thigh against the bed frame and inner-spring mattress—then tug, pull, and tuck for whatever results you want to achieve.

Caution: Since you will be doing the above tug 'n' tuck maneuvers without your crutches—in order to bend down low enough as well as to keep your hands free—adequate balance and strength are required. If they are still in short supply, station a chair nearby and sit instead to make the bed.

12 Clothing: Getting It On and Getting It Off

Whether it's hip replacement or Achilles tendon repair you're stuck with, managing basic daily functions in the least time- and energy-consuming manner possible is primarily a matter of thinking out things in advance. That means organization.

It takes practice, and while you're learning there will be moments of utter frustration when you've forgotten something vital and only you will fully comprehend your wasted time and energy—and what that means to a person who can barely get around. (*No one* else will really understand—you have to get used to that.)

So the "biggies" in conquering the woes of dressing are Organization and Time. Time—plan on extra, perhaps lots extra. Later on, as you get more experienced, you can cut down.

● ● ●Word to the Wise: APPEARANCE. To feel good it helps to look good. Now's not the time to neglect personal appearance. Looking good can raise your morale when coping with the frustrations of a clumsy or useless leg. Those around you will benefit too.

Types of Clothing

Loose-fitting clothes—"sweats" are a perfect example—are easiest for getting on and off when dealing with a cast, non-weight-bearing status, and most types of leg injury and surgery.

Pants and skirts: Pants or skirts with elastic waists and no zippers or buttons to battle are less complicated in getting on and also in arranging. Since dressing chores take place at least twice a day—many more if you include putting on clothes for the outdoors, changing for a workout, and other activities—energy conservation is important. Pleated or loose skirts and comfortably sized dresses are easier than tight ones when you're using crutches, as long as they are not so commodious as to get in the way. Pants legs can be cut along the seam and, for long-term cast immobilization, be zippered or have Velcro tabs attached. Pants with full-length side zippers are available from camping outfitters.

Pullover shirts and sweaters: Such garments are practical because they are easily slipped on over the head, and there are no buttons to strain and pop or openings to sag. Shirts or blouses with long shirt tails that will stay tucked in are good, although women may want to avoid front-opening apparel which—as they use, or rest, on their crutches—can reveal more than they desire.

Suspenders: Stretchy suspenders are useful because they don't let pants slip down as your upper body contorts with crutches. They're much easier and quicker than belts, which can be an advantage when getting to the toilet is so time-consuming. Women find suspenders practical too.

Jewelry: Bracelets and watches can get damaged or broken when worn in conjunction with crutch use.

Bed clothes: Getting comfy in bed is hard with a cast to heave around and weakened muscles to do it with. If you have them, fabrics that slide easily are best.

Keeping warm: Feeling cold is natural if you're not moving around a lot. If you are non-weight-bearing, the toes—or the whole leg if it's uncasted—are especially vulnerable. Layering is the answer: light garments that can easily be put on or taken off as needed. Nowadays there is winter underwear that has no bulk whatsoever—including lightweight silks that can go under anything from leisure clothes to suits and dresses—and which agreeably counteracts the walrus look that three sweaters and two sets of pants would create. The injured leg, if it's uncasted, can be individually layered in whatever combination works for you: knee-high hose, knee socks, leg warmers, thin socks, thick socks, even gaiters—there's gear galore.

Fabrics: Wear easy-care, permanent-press fabrics to cut down on laundry time, an essential consideration in your life right now. Lightweight materials are energy savers both in getting clothing on and off as well as in the wearing. Lastly, remove clothes from the dryer immediately so wrinkles and ironing are lessened.

Aids to Dressing and Undressing

Dressing chair: Have a sturdy, stable chair that will serve as the center of your dressing area. It should be easy to get down to and up from, not a soft and low easy chair. It might well be the straight-backed chair that is in your bathroom (see Chapter 10).

Bed: Your bed is an alternative dressing area. A drawback is that you are not centralized at the bathroom-sink location where so many grooming tasks are performed — a saving on energy used getting from place to place. An advantage, however — for some people — is that the bed can make dressing easier. In this case, they put pants legs on over each foot, then lie on their back to pull up lower-body garments while using their good foot and leg to raise their hips. See below for more detailed suggestions on streamlining dressing drudgery.

Table: A table near your dressing area, preferably with extra shelves, is ideal for stacking of frequently used clothes, makeup and personal-grooming needs.

Reacher: A wire coat hanger — stretched apart with the hook end retained — is useful for many dressing chores, from pulling up pants over a casted leg to reaching hard-to-get items. If you've a cane in your life, it can be useful in many of the same ways.

Undressing

Positioning: Stand next to your dressing-area chair, stabilizing yourself with the outside of your calf pressed against it in the manner explained in Chapter 7.

"Drop artist": Drop all your lower-body garments around your ankles — your pants or skirt, and then your underwear, *without* sitting down between garments — an energy-saving lack of movement.

Sitting: Now sit down and remove the shoe, then the sock, the pants leg, and underwear leg in that order from the good limb followed by the injured one. (The uninjured leg is done first because it can be more easily bent and manipulated for removal of clothes.) Taking everything off one leg before doing the other leg is both an energy- and a time-saver. Take off upper-body duds next.

• • •Word to the Wise: NEAT AND TIDY. It will be easier on you if you learn from the very beginning not to discard those duds all over the floor, because picking them up is a chore you definitely want to avoid. Do necessary folding while you're sitting and undressing. If any of the garments are to be worn the next day, of course, to save time and energy do not put them away in closets or drawers. Place them nearby for quick retrieval.

It is pretty obvious that dressing will be the reverse of undressing; however, there are a number of important differences which will affect the amount of time you spend. Since you'll want to preserve maximum morning sack time, better read on.

Preparation: Organize. Choose your clothes and shoes, and place them next to your dressing chair. For how to get your clothes there, see below as well as Chapter 14.

Positioning: Seat yourself; establish your crutches nearby.

Upper-body put-on: The upper body gets garbed first, so it's on with your undershirt or bra, shirt and tie, dress or blouse, sweater or jacket—everything, including jewelry. If you have your makeup and toiletries properly organized—mirror, brush, deodorant, aftershave, lipstick, etc.—they are nearby in a small basket or other container. Now is the time to use them while you are sitting down and before you start draping your legs with unwieldy garments.

Caution: When pulling garments over your head—whether putting on or taking off—make sure you are either sitting down or leaning against a sturdy and steady object such as a bureau or wall. Balance is extremely poor when you are teetering on one leg and your eyes are covered by a garment.

Partial lower-body pull-up: The lower bod comes next. The injured leg is done first, since garments can be put on it without needing to drastically bend it. Underwear, then socks or panty hose if used, followed by shorts or pants or skirt. All these things get pulled up as far as possible while you are sitting down. Now your shoes—and tie them so you don't trip. (See above, on dressing while using your bed instead of a dressing chair.)

Note: If a full-length cast prevents you from easily bending down and tying your shoe, there are elastic laces available that remain tied and stretch so you can push your foot into the shoe. Shoes with Velcro tabs are another solution to this problem. Specialized sock and stocking aids can also be helpful in coping with an inflexible leg. See Chapter 19 for details.

Stand up: Use your crutches to help you stand up, as explained in Chapter 7. Establish them nearby, and stabilize yourself appropriately against the chair or bed with the angled-leg technique.

Finish of pull-up: The clothing that has accumulated somewhere in the vicinity of your knees now needs to be pulled up the rest of the way in logical order. Tucking in and straightening would be a good idea too.

Order! Organization!

You now see that dressing and undressing can be relatively quick processes if done in the above sequences, but without the clothes at hand you'll be constantly struggling to stand up and fetch them, resulting in wasted time and corresponding fatigue and frustration. Getting up and down unnecessarily is a real strain that the limp-and-gimp set should avoid.

So, one by one, get your clothing needs to your designated dressing area, laying them out if possible on a nearby table or chair. If you're a workin' dude, it's best to lay out the duds the night before, all the way to such accessories as jewelry, purse, tie, belt, and handkerchief.

TOTIN', TUGGIN', HEAVIN', 'N' HAULIN'

Although there is a separate chapter on the many challenging aspects of this subject (see Chapter 14), a start will be made right now for the specialized requirements of the "robing department."

Let's admit immediately how annoying and frustrating it is (you'll have that feeling often) to get your clothes from where they're stored — whether a closet or bureau in your room or somewhere else even less convenient — to your designated dressing area. To carry a dress or suit on a hanger while clutching and stumbling along on crutches seems like a tall order indeed. (In fact, the taller you are the better — for the garment in question is less likely to drag on the floor.)

The long and the short of it is that coping with each closet or bureau and each type of garment almost has to be figured out individually. But, you *can* manage on your own; here are a few tips to help.

Caution: Many of the techniques to carry clothes are advanced, requiring good balance and reasonable skill with crutches.

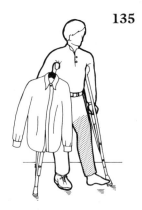

There are several ways to manage clothes on hangers: take your choice.

Armpit-pad hanger-hitch: Place the hanger loop over the armpit pad of your crutch on the stronger side, and just crutch along. The length of the garment makes this carry awkward, but it works.

Handgrip hanger-hitch: Hitch the hanger loop over the handgrip on the stronger side crutch and — ditto, step along. You have a little better control, except that the garment — unless it's a jacket, blouse, or skirt — generally drags. (At this point sometimes you just don't care.)

Teeth clutch: If you're not afraid of ruining your All-American smile — and the garment is a short one — take the hanger in your teeth and move along that way. It's often the easiest and quickest method of them all and useful for many other quick carries — especially if you don't mind that your public will think you're demonstrating fetching to a golden retriever.

Shirts, Sweaters, and Other Garments Not on Hangers

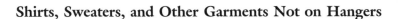

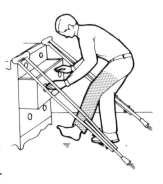

As usual with anything you are removing from a closet or bureau, those confounded crutches have to be established near at hand and ideally where they won't fall — so you don't have to pick them up as well.

For bureaus place the *armpit pads* (not the handgrips) of the crutches against the top edge or a drawer edge depending on its size, one on either side of you — the crutch tips will be a-ground behind you. This positions the crutches almost horizontal to the floor, making it possible to open the drawer. The rubber pads keep them from sliding. Your balance is secured by holding on to the bureau or by the action of pulling on the drawer.

To carry garments without hangers, use the methods below:

Hand and grip clutch: Use the hand on the strong side to clutch both the handgrip of the crutch and the article of clothing.

Neck drape: Drape clothing around your neck or over your shoulder. (Are you a "clothes horse," or what?)

Teeth toting: If you're using crutches, your teeth will constantly be called upon to help. As there's not much chance of damaging them ivories on cloth, feel free.

Tossin' and throwin':   To add a bit of excitement to the drab duty of dragging duds, it should be pointed out that you can "shoot" items of clothing — or anything else — once you are in range of where you are taking them. At this stage of your crutch life it can be one of life's very small but satisfying feelings to hit a target, make that shot, score that goal. Laundry basket or washing machine, dressing chair or bed — innovate. Remember, however, that minor misses mean major retrieval — balance energy dissipation against psychic inspiration.

Flipping out: The strong-side crutch tip can also be employed to create diversion, such as propelling dirty laundry to a hamper and other contests still to be invented. When you're feeling sassy and adventurous, go for flipping garments airborne toward the "net" — it may not be a slam dunk, but it's a vote for a little bit of frolic during these days of life in the slow lane. (And who knows? These games may have a fantastic future — so create, and earn yourself a place in history.)

Footwear

Shoe transportation is another matter entirely — heaving them where they need to go can almost be labeled easy or fun. Somehow you get a feeling of being in charge, for once, and that's a charge you don't often get when you're learning to hobble around after a metal plate has been screwed into your tibia or your ligament has been replaced. Anyway, shoes lend themselves admirably to the "shot on goal" system — and if your shoe on goal misses, use the tip of the strong-side crutch to hook them in the heel and heave them onward.

● ● ●Words to the Wise for Women: DRESSES AND BLOUSES. Be aware of your dresses or blouses that have necks or collars with wide or low openings. Walking with crutches or leaning over and resting on your crutches may make your clothing more revealing than you desire. JEWELRY: Do not wear loose or dangling bracelets. They get damaged or broken by being constantly caught between your wrist and the crutch. A wrist watch, unless covered by apparel, is at risk as well.

Dressing for the Outdoors: Coats and Jackets

Dressing accomplished, you may want to go out. Colder weather makes this a bit more burdensome — more clothes to cope with — but the technique which follows will keep the frustration factor under control.

The key to sophisticated coating or jacketing is to position yourself against a wall, sturdy piece of furniture, or counter. Balance yourself properly, then establish the crutches nearby. You're now set to put on whatever is required in a stable and secure manner, without having to cling to some well-meaning but inexperienced acquaintance or totter dangerously on your own.

Presto. Before you even know it, you are sheathed against the elements with little fuss or waste of energy.

13   Coping in the Kitchen

Such tasks as are implied in the above title are pretty awesome under-takings when you are hobbled in any way by leg problems, much less using a walker or crutches. Each and every step of meal-preparation has suddenly been transformed from "ho-hum" and taken for granted to laborious and extremely time-consuming. Even advanced, long-term crutch users will probably hold back from big-time cooking unless they have an unusually helpful and understanding assistant. (If there is a choice, having the crutch user be the assistant is of course, wiser and more realistic. And, unless you have time and will power to spare— plan on simple fare.)

But, as always, there's more than one way to skin a cat, and although it's to be hoped no such cuisine figures in your kitchen, here are some suggestions to make feeding less of a fight for a crutch-wielding cook. Others in recovery—whether their status is partial-weight-bearing, advanced limping, or cane coping—will find hunger pangs easier to avoid as well.

A for Apron and B for Basket: Indispensable Accessories

As pointed out in Chapter 2, if there is any one, simple, unexotic, inexpensive, and utilitarian object that will make your life infinitely easier and more independent, the getting-back-on-your-feet apron may be it. Baskets and basket-carts rank right up there too, because of all the food—cooked and uncooked—or plates or glasses or utensils— clean and dirty—that you'll be totin'.

Please turn rapidly, swiftly, and without delay—meaning now— to Chapter 14 to find out how a simple apron and basket can make such a difference. (The kitchen is a place you'll need to know your ABC's, for sure.)

If neither your apron nor a rolling basket-cart is available, what do you do to get food items and utensils from one area of the kitchen to another? Although modern kitchen design minimizes such hurdles, it is not the size of the kitchen that is the hardship so much as it is the problem of transferring heavy or unwieldy objects any distance at all.

> *Caution:* If the objects to be carried are either very heavy or very hot, the following maneuver becomes advanced technique and is *not* suitable for beginners or persons with shaky balance. An essential skill to have already mastered is the armpit grip, by which you hold one crutch with the muscles of the upper arm and free a hand for other duties.

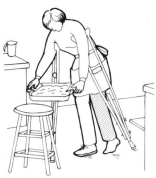

Chair, table, or bar stool "transfer station":   Place a chair, bar stool, or any small table—a spare bedside table would do—in the center of the kitchen to establish a way station between facilities. Unwieldy objects from one kitchen area are moved to the desired area via this station. Thus, a heavy bowl or gallon of milk would be moved from the fridge directly to the way station (chair, stool, or whatever) and from there over to the sink, food-preparation area, or stove. A heavy saucepan might be transferred from the sink via table station to the stove and—if you have heat-resistant surfaces—a hot casserole might go from oven to stool station to counter.

The crafty combination of a way station with a skillful armpit grip gives *lots* of opportunities to function on your own and impress friends and family with your coping mechanisms and independence.

Kitchen Counters as Transfer Stations

Any flat surfaces in a kitchen are built-in way stations for food, plates, or utensils—counter top, stove top, or top of a fridge.

Get pushy: Push pots or plates on those surfaces as far as you're able, pick them up and move them on to the next surface available, and so on—until you have gotten the item to where you want it to go or the counter has run out on you. Then use any of the other methods to get the object to its designated place, whether it is the dining table for eating or the cupboard for storage.

D for Definitely Needed Rest Spot

A counter-height chair, bar stool, adjustable chair, or stool of almost any kind is a highly recommended addition to your kitchen work area—not only for its transferral possibilities, but so you can sit or perch on it while preparing meals. If it possesses a seat back and a foot rest, all the better.

A working-area seat not only conserves overall energy but also your *uninjured* foot and leg—which will frequently rebel at lengthy sessions of peeling, chopping, or watching pots coming to a boil. Possibilities are a secretary's or executive's chair—the office-type chair that swivels, rolls, and is adjustable in height—or a medical-style examining stool, both of which can also be used for elevation of your injured leg when you're sitting elsewhere. By all means, obtain some sort of elevated seat, and save some vim, vigor, and vitality to enjoy what you cooked and any company you are sharing it with.

Storage and Reaching

For the duration of your recovery, you will avoid being the fastidious individual you may or may not have always been. You don't have to be a slob, but you will not be putting things away that you use frequently. Items that are normally stored out of reach will reside on your counter top or some other accessible spot. If you're temporarily in a wheelchair, get items relocated to lower shelves in the refrigerator and freezer if possible, as well as elsewhere in the kitchen. Use a hanger, cane, cut-off hockey stick, or other homemade invention to help with reaching and pulling. Reachers that can grab and hold items instead of just poking or pulling are available from medical-supply stores or through mail order (see Chapter 19).

Kitchen Potpourri

Sink spray hose: If your sink is adjacent to the stove, place empty pots on the stove and fill them with the spray hose right where they sit.

Caution: If you are using crutches, a wheelchair, or walker, be careful when reaching to the back of a stove across active burners and pots cooking on the front. Your reach is shorter, and your stability is lessened. Long-handled barbecue tools can be used for stirring and lifting items of food.

Hospital-style, over-bed table: This type of table is also very useful in a kitchen, giving you an adjustable-height surface which can go over your lap for preparing foods, eating, and chores of many sorts, all while you're sitting down with your injured leg properly elevated. It is also an ideal way station because of its wheels and adjustability. See Chapter 19 for a mail-order source.

Saving energy: To conserve strength, do every household chore sitting down if possible. This includes work in the laundry, where a chair should be placed for jobs like folding clothes. Ironing, if unable to be eliminated, should be done from a high-seated kitchen stool or chair, preferably one on casters.

Try to alternate tiring tasks with lighter ones to keep your energy from being depleted. Be on the lookout for more efficient ways to do chores that cannot be delegated or avoided altogether.

Tongs: Long-handled barbecue tongs are handy in reaching stuff you've dropped on the floor—saving energy and frustration—as well as clutching packages, cans of food, and miscellaneous objects in countless other situations.

Clean-up: Utilize your smarts to save on energy and time-consuming clean-up. Shop at places that sell frozen, prepared, or partially prepared foods, from pizza parlors to salad bars to fancy meat counters with ready-to-cook entrees. Prepare fresh food with throwaway paper towels underneath—to catch juices, parings, peelings, and the like. Use nonstick cookware. Store leftovers that are microwavable in containers that can go in the microwave directly from the refrigerator without a change.

Double portions: Prepare double portions of whatever you make. Serve one and freeze or refrigerate the other for another meal. Extensive variety in meal offerings is not a consideration when you're recovering from foot fracture, hip replacement, or anything in between.

Delivery: If a grocery store in your area delivers, consider using their service at least for the first few difficult days. Or have someone do a major marketing—good for two weeks or so—at a supermarket, and use the delivery-service store for perishables and "forgottens." As you won't be lured into impulse buying at the supermarket, the cost may not be all that different.

Marketing: To save energy and time, go to the market that carries the greatest number of goods you need—and preferably one that provides help with packing and loading your car.

• • •Word to the Wise: LEVEL PARKING. A level parking lot is very important for getting in and out of your car — for safety, for as little fatigue as possible, and for ease of loading.

Avoid marketing at peak periods — lunchtime and after work — when possible. Arrange your marketing list before you go, with items grouped by where they are located. If you get tired easily, the list might be planned in order of priority instead — so that the most important items are in hand if you are unable to finish shopping.

If possible, also organize the grocery cart. Have four bags in it, placing frozen items in one, refrigerator items in another, staples and canned goods in the third, and cleaning supplies in the last one.

Difficulty in opening doors in kitchen area: Weakness and instability can make even commonplace appliance or cupboard doors a challenge. If your freezer or fridge leaves you frazzled, place a piece of electrical or duct tape across the door gasket in one or two places to break the vacuum seal. It will result in a slight loss of energy efficiency but a gain in yours — which is more important at this moment of your life. If you're using a wheelchair or crutches, cupboard doors, screen doors, or any door can have a strap looped to the handle to ease some of the difficulty by allowing you to position yourself farther away. Leverage is increased and opening radius improved.

Fetch and Carry   14

The tips you pick up in this chapter will make a real difference between being self-sufficient and independent, or just the opposite: constantly asking someone (who's probably busy or would prefer not to be disturbed) to fetch or carry something for you. Absorb the basic and advanced techniques which follow, and before long you'll be creating your own inventive solutions for your own unique situations.

A IS FOR APRON

For women *and men* equally, this may be the single most valuable tip you will get from this book in terms of self-sufficiency, independence, and even safety. Explanations follow, but *now* — make an apron, get someone else to make you one, or alter one so that it will fit the specifications outlined below. The pockets are the key to carrying, and the apron carries *them*. It's simple, and it's essential, and you'll soon see why.

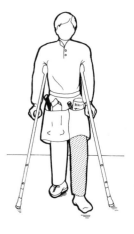

Uses: Anything that fits those apron pockets can be carried: reading material, writing materials, portable phone, magazines, the newspaper, food, beverages, crockery, tools — *anything*. And indoors or outdoors, upstairs or downstairs — anywhere.

One of the biggest difficulties for a leg-injured person is preparing meals. The transportation of items needed for meals from the various storage areas — refrigerator, freezer, cupboards, and the like — to the preparation area, and vice versa, is the hardest part of that. The apron and its pockets are the way to go. From fruit or freezer fare to the fixings for a stew, you (and your apron) will be fetching like a kangaroo.

You can certainly visualize now how much more self-sufficient you will be if you can get what you want from one place to another without resorting to ouside help, or precariously hopping with food and utensils awkwardly clutched in the single finger you can spare from the crutch or walker itself. Mentally multiply all the trips you need in

143

the preparation of a single dish—not to mention an entire meal or to complete chores of any kind—and the lowly apron becomes a real saver—a saver of your strength, your time, and your sanity.

Safety:　Improved safety results from the simple fact that in using the apron you won't be using other, more precarious forms of transportation. But by far the most substantial increase in safety lies in the fact that with the apron, the weight you are transporting is centered solidly in front of you, where you and it are balanced more effectively.

Items or bags of any kind carried or dangled from a crutch hand do more than just unbalance you to one side—they swing forward in front of the crutch as you move, preventing normal progression and encouraging a fall.

Adapting or Making Your Apron

Material:　The material should be as sturdy as it would be in any store-bought apron and can be any that you have on hand.

Bib:　The apron need not have a bib that covers the chest and ties behind the neck, unless you prefer. (If so, it can have a small, additional pocket put there.) In general, however, the bib adds another onerous chore of putting on as well as tying something—at a time when you're already struggling with a lot of other frustrations. So, if you're altering an existing apron, you can cut the bib portion off.

Pockets:　The crucial requirement is that the apron have two large pockets firmly attached; 13 by 12 inches is a convenient and workable size. The itty-bitty pockets that aprons normally have are not sufficient for the large variety of items you will be transporting in them. Cut off those "itty-bitties" and sew on "he-man" pockets.

Now—that's all the reasoning and explanations that any doubter deserves: wear your apron, wear it because you're smart—and smart enough not to be too proud to wear it.

B IS FOR BASKET (OR BASKET-CART)

A is for Apron is for guys 'n' gals at home: with lots of chores to do, maybe with a few kids underfoot—maybe just trying to cope any way at all. While B for Basket is also for serious household involvement, it is even more practical for those in businesses and stores with lots of paper or products to push. The basket should be on wheels, of course, and options include the small supermarket type, a serving cart, or department-store and mail-order models that have plastic storage bins. A castered table with several shelves is also extremely helpful—especially at chair or bedside for business being conducted at home as well as for general use.

> *Caution:* When you're moving any wheeled cart or table, keep your weight centered on your crutches, not on the cart or table. Push it ahead, then catch up; don't let it pull you into a fall.

OTHER WAYS OF CARRYING THINGS

Wagon

If you are faced with bringing groceries, packages, or anything a long distance outside, a child's wagon might be a solution. However, your balance and strength must be good and your crutch techniques advanced enough to permit using the armpit grip (see below for precise explanation).

Teeth

Odd as it may sound and look, using one's teeth to carry small items is the first way that comes to mind in the "dawn of one's crutch life." Letters, a piece of clothing, a paperback book, a bag of potato chips—the list is endless. Even when you're in the "twilight" of your crutch life, it's a good bet you'll still be using your ivories—though by then you'll have mastered a multitude of more advanced methods.

Pocket or Waistband Tuck

Basic—as well as obvious—is your pocket for whatever you can stuff into it. Less obvious, the waistband of your skirt or pants is also handy, offering a casual and temporary substitute for the apron. Tuck in a wallet, newspaper, hat, or whatever else you need for a limited jaunt, and off you go.

Shopping Bags, Paper Bags

Aprons are not a popular item of attire outside the home, so if you are appearance-conscious you have to make do with some awkward substitutes when you go outside. Shopping bags are easier to hold on to than plain paper bags because of the handles, but a major drawback is that they swing in front of the crutch as you move along. Proceed cautiously.

If a plain paper bag is available, get one that is overlarge, big enough to fold down the top into a roll that you can grip securely while also holding on to the handgrip of your crutch. This type of bag will not swing in front, allowing you to walk much more easily as well as faster.

Packs and Bags

Day pack or backpack: If you want to swing along in relative freedom and also carry quite a bit, a day pack — a very small version of the hiker's backpack — is the answer. It is also a solution for the businessman or woman who will have trouble handling his or her normal briefcase. Adaptations of such packs are sold as student book bags, making them ideal not only for the student who has broken a leg skiing but also for the executive who wishes he *hadn't* gone skiing and broken his leg. These packs are found in camping outlets and department stores.

Fanny pack or tummy pack: Fanny packs are zippered pouches of various sizes that belt around your waist. They hold less than the day pack but are adequate for most needs, as well as being easier to put on and use. Although they are called "fanny" packs, they can just as easily be worn in front. Find them where day packs are sold.

Tote bag: This type of bag is a practical option only if it has straps long enough to be swung over your head onto the far shoulder. Your balance is not compromised as long as the bag is kept pushed around to the back. The drawback is that this needs to be done frequently.

Purse, handbag: A woman's purse presents the same problems that a shopping bag or other normally handheld item does. It's easily solved, though, by carrying the type with long skinny straps which can be slung over your head onto the far shoulder like the tote bag mentioned above. Also like the tote bag, this kind of purse will have to be kept pushed back onto your posterior. Keep it smallish, and if you're accustomed to carrying everything but the kitchen sink, jettison all but the essentials.

Traveling light while on crutches saves energy for getting places. On some occasions you may be able to get by with just sticking cash or credit card, comb, and lipstick into a skirt or slacks pocket. For security reasons, do this in high-risk areas anyway; persons hampered by mobility aids need to take extra precautions. The "up side" is that with nothing at all slung over shoulder or hung from crutches "get-up-and-go" urges are more readily heeded.

PUSHING, PULLING, AND LIFTING: CRUTCHES AS HELPMATES

There are some simple ways, as well as some esoteric ones, in which crutches can either be employed as accessories or manipulated in advanced techniques that free up a hand for a projected task. (Canes are no slouches, either, in the helpmate department.)

Push, Poke, and Pull

At the very beginning of your crutch life you'll soon find yourself using one crutch to support yourself and the other to push things in the direction you want them to go or to pull them to you. Something in your way? Take the crutch and swat the object to another, preferred location. No doubt it'll take several swats, but you'll have done it without having to wait for someone else. Dropped something? Pull it toward you with your rubber-tipped tool. Ensconced comfortably and the door needs shutting? Give it a poke with that extra-long appendage you're traveling around with. The possibilities are endless.

Lifting and Heaving

This gets into a bit more advanced technique because better balance is required, but both the balance and the strength to go with it are soon acquired. If you need to lift a firm-sided object, such as a carton, the trick is to employ the crutches like chopsticks or tongs. You pinch the item between the crutch tips and lift it quickly over a door lintel, a stair lip, or the edge of a rug, for example, so that you can continue poking and pushing it in the way described above.

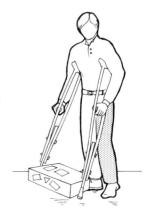

> ***Caution:*** At the point of lifting you are without tripod stability, so your balance and crutch skills must be good. The moment, however, is brief, and by the time you are up to advanced tricks like this, it won't seem precarious at all.

FETCHING AND CARRYING ON CRUTCHES

Basic Armpit Grip

This advanced technique has been described before; if you've not learned it yet, adopt it right now instead of undergoing additional weeks of being more dependent on others than you might wish. One of

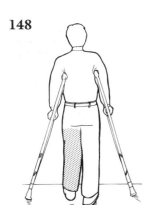

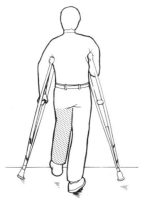

the most satisfying actions it will allow you to accomplish on your own is carrying a comforting mug of coffee or tea whenever *you* want—as opposed to when someone else is free to bring you one.

The armpit grip differs from standard crutching in that instead of using your hand to help hold the strong-side crutch, the crutch is only held by the muscles of the upper arm in conjunction with the elbow, leaving the hand on that side free to carry an object.

Positioning: Use the normal tripod position to start.

Weak-side crutch grip: The hand holds the handgrip as is normal on the injured-leg side.

Strong-side armpit grip: Grip the crutch with the muscles of the armpit, upper arm, and elbow. The hand does not hold on to the handgrip.

Crutch carry: The strong-side crutch, in this method, will be *hitched* directly forward by the armpit-arm-elbow grip.

> *Note:* Since you are not holding on to the crutch with your hand, your weight will now be supported at your armpit on the axillary pad of the crutch, contrary to the method recommended for standard crutching. However, as armpit-grip techniques are used only for specialized tasks of short duration, there is little risk of nerve damage. When employed early in your crutch life, the grip may make your armpit feel a little tender; time will toughen it. (With most ankle, knee, or leg injuries time—minimally eight weeks worth—is something you have.)

Advanced Armpit Grip

This is a refinement to try after you have mastered the basic armpit grip, above.

Positioning: Use the normal tripod position.

Weak-side crutch grip: The hand holds the handgrip in the normal way.

Strong-side armpit grip: Grip the crutch with the muscles of the armpit, upper arm, and elbow. The hand does not hold on to the handgrip.

Bump and grind: The crutch, in this method, will not be hitched directly forward by the armpit grip. Instead, direct the elbow and crutch *diagonally in front of your body* as you take a step—while at the same time giving the crutch added impetus and forward motion

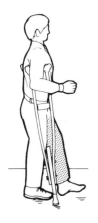 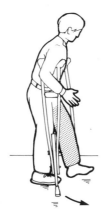 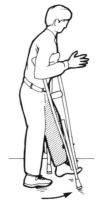

with a good push by the hip. The hip-shove bumps the crutch forward at an angle. This subtle and sophisticated maneuver enables you to move a greater distance with each hop—as well as faster—while at the same time keeping a hand free. With advantages such as those—not to mention how professional you'll look—this is obviously a technique worth acquiring.

Pinkie Grip

This method is a compromise between the normal full-hand grip and the armpit-elbow grip described above. The pinkie grip is useful and fast for carrying an object of a weight and design that permits your hand to be used both to carry the object *and* move the crutch at the same time. A coffee mug is a good example—lightweight and with a handle. Give it a try as follows:

Positioning: Use the normal tripod position to start.

Weak-side crutch grip: The hand holds the handgrip in the normal way.

Strong-side armpit grip: Grip the crutch with the muscles of the armpit, upper arm, and elbow.

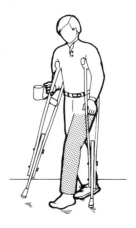

Pinkie grip: The hand does not hold on to the handgrip. Instead the fifth (pinkie) finger is looped around the *leading* edge of the crutch at the normal handgrip level. The pinkie then pulls the crutch along and forward with the help of the armpit hitch while the thumb and the remaining fingers of that hand are free for transporting. A bit of the hip-generated bump and grind that is used in advanced armpit skills—described above—helps too. You are still able to maintain fairly good forward momentum, which of course is the name of the game—if you're stuck on sticks.

Moving Large, Heavy Objects via the Tortoise Approach

This method demonstrates how the approach used by Aesop's fabled tortoise—patient determination—conquers not only boastful hares but most everything else as well. Generally speaking, an effort of this sort will be to lift an object from the floor or ground—such as a bag of groceries you want to get in from the car or a briefcase to your desk.

Positioning: Place both crutches under the weak-side armpit, making sure you are well balanced.

Bend "zee" leg: Bend your strong leg, lean down, grab hold of whatever needs to be moved, and lift it a bit in the direction you want it to go.

> *Caution:* Normal back precautions are difficult to observe when doing this lift. Avoid it altogether if you have back problems.

Repositioning: Replace your crutches in their usual walking position, hop to the parcel, get both crutches under one arm again, and repeat the small lift.

Repeat: The above gets repeated until the mission is accomplished. Slow like a tortoise, indeed—and although you won't win any races you will have gotten to the finish line.

> *Caution:* This is an advanced technique, requiring good crutch skills, good balance, and adequate strength.

Heaving Objects Upstairs via the Tortoise Approach

The tortoise technique described above is also used for getting objects, large or small, upstairs. To go for it, here's how.

Positioning: Position yourself and the object to be lifted at the bottom of the stairs. Place both crutches under the weak-side armpit.

Bend and toss: Bend down and lift or toss the object to the highest tread you can reach.

Repositioning: Replace the crutches in their normal position and ascend to the stair within reaching distance of the object.

Repeat: Put both crutches back under the weak-side armpit, bend once more, toss once more.

Slow? Yes. Successful? Yes. 'Nuff said? Yes.

> *Caution:* Because of the difficult nature of stairs in general, any maneuver on them is considered advanced, requiring good crutch skills and excellent balance.

Hauling, Pushing, and Pulling

To move or bring an object toward you—a heavy armchair or car door, for instance—or to push it away, there are a couple of minor departures from the lifting and heaving techniques described above.

Positioning: Have your crutches in the normal location, under each armpit, for strong and sturdy support. Place yourself within reaching distance, but not too close, to the object to be moved.

Armpit grip: You'll be using the armpit grip on both sides so that both your hands are freed, or only one side if that's all you need.

Pull: Now haul. Repeat all steps as necessary.

Use the same strategy to push heavy objects away from you.

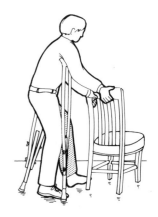

Picking Up Objects

There's hardly anything more frustrating for the individual coping with injury and mobility aids than the seemingly innocuous and simple task of retrieving items that have been dropped or that somehow have ended up on the floor or ground. On each occasion you have to settle your crutches against some stable surface, rearrange your equilibrium, and then do ye olde balancing act to repossess that tool, that fork, that hat, that whatever. During the course of a normal day the staunchest spirit can feel like emitting more than the occasional scream. To keep those at a minimum, here are a few hints.

Seated retrieval: A complicated orthopaedic operation and bed rest can leave you too shaky and pooped for many of the maneuvers that follow. Here's one that will fill the gap. If feasible, push or pull a chair close to the object to be picked up, sit down, and then pick it up. There will be no problems with balance or safety, and after retrieving the item you can rest before proceeding.

Basic standing retrieval: With all retrievals, the first thing to do is to establish your crutches somewhere. In the basic or normal method this means leaning them against a counter, bureau, chair, workbench, vehicle, or other stable surface. Lean them with the rubber armpits or handgrips against that surface so they will not slide to the floor, avoiding—hallelujah—another pickup. Finally, hold on to that stable surface, bend down, and pick up whatever it is that has fallen.

Advanced standing retrieval: If you are in the middle of no-where, so to speak — a driveway, field, airport terminal, parking lot, or whatever — the challenge is to both pick up the object *and* keep hold of your crutches when there is no place to establish them. There's no need to panic — read on for enabling tactics.

Remove both crutches from their armpit locations and hold them by the paired handgrips in your weak-side hand, their tips a-ground. No weight at all will be supported by the crutches as you hold the crutches out to the side — tips on the ground — directly in line with, but out and away from the weak-side limb. The crutch tips must be grounded far enough away so that they allow you to get in "retrieval position" — which means the arm holding the crutches will be stretched horizontally away from the body.

Then — get set, bend the good knee, and down you go. The crutches will go down too — almost flat out — and all your weight will be on your good leg. A spectacular retrieve — performed by a true and certified crutchjock.

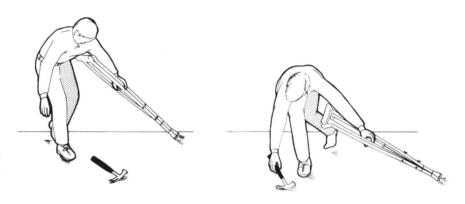

Caution: Warning repeated that this is advanced stuff, since there is absolutely no tripod security at a time when a major maneuver is being performed. Excellent balance and adequate good-leg strength, as well as adequate good-knee range of motion are required. The same warnings apply to the retrievals that follow.

Advanced retrieval, a variation: For a casual, laid-back retrieve, a casual, laid-back place to park the spare crutch is — instead of against a counter or tree — right against your midriff. Intrigued? — details follow.

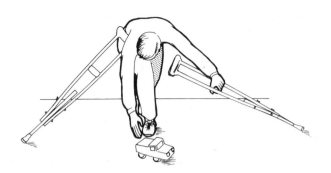

In this method, hold only the weak-side crutch out to the side as described and place the other directly *in front* or to the strong side of your body, rubber head perching against your midriff. (You can even lean *both* crutches against your midsection.) Once again you've got a hand (or hands) freed up for retrieving, and the utter simplicity of the gambit will indelibly mark you—especially to other cognoscenti—as a sophisticate of crutch life.

Advanced retrieval, another variation: In this method, the weak-side crutch is turned on its side and, at the place where it balances properly, is grasped by its wooden extension and kept next to the hip rather than laying it out to the side. (The crutch tip will be out behind you and the armpit bar out in front of you.) The strong-side crutch is established against your midriff or pelvic joint (see above). As there is no tripod support, you will dip quickly on your good leg, do the retrieve, and then resume the normal tripod position.

15 Cooling Cabin Fever and Making Time Fly: Getting Places, Recreation, Travel

Physical restriction of any sort—whether due to a cast, knee reconstruction, a broken toe, or anything else—makes most people feel frustrated and angry. Restriction is imprisonment—and the result can be acute cabin fever. Suddenly most normal activities have been denied—or those activities have become enormously difficult to accomplish. With every single act so time-consuming and burdensome, it's not surprising that the majority of newly injured withdraw from involvements—and thus cut themselves off from the persons they usually see at work, sports, or social engagements.

Weariness pervades because low levels of activity make body systems drag. Emptiness pervades because the self is thinking inwardly the "Why" Syndrome ("Why did this have to happen to me?") or the "Woe" Syndrome ("Woe is me: think of all I'm missing.").

There is really nothing anyone else can do about such a dilemma, the dilemma of filling time. It is up to you to find resources within yourself—and without—to take on the challenges and make the most of the days ahead, even to the point of capitalizing on them as the precious commodity they are—"found time."

One way is to use the skills already described, and the others which follow, to *get out and go*. This period of restricted living will present all sorts of opportunities—for activities that there has not been time for previously, for cultivating new friendships and re-establishing old ones, for excursions and trips of many kinds. Don't let time drag, get up and go.

CARS AND DRIVING

> *Caution:* Get your doctor's permission before you hit the wide-open road.

Left-leg injury: For starters, we'll just have to accept as a given that you're in luck if the injured limb or foot is the left one. That makes driving easy—at least eas-i-er—if you have a vehicle with an automatic transmission. But if all you have is a gear-shifting vehicle and if you desire to be independent, there's no doubt about it—you'll just have to borrow, rent, or steal a car with an automatic transmission. For country dwellers especially—wheels are a must in the fight against cabin fever.

Right-leg injury: Those with right-leg problems need to import an English vehicle quick—or learn to drive with the left leg. Yes, it can be done—it is done—but don't venture out on the open road cold turkey. Practicing first—in your driveway or on a quiet street—is recommended. To be extra law-abiding, you might check to see if local ordinances prohibit such innovations. If your injury will make driving dicey for a long time to come, there are easily installed driving aids such as left foot accelerators. See Chapter 19 on where to obtain them.

If your right leg is the injured one, get in the car on the *passenger's side* and slide over to the driver's seat. Then, without any strain to get it there, you can just *leave* the bum leg lying over the driveshaft hump. It will be kept out of the way and—more to the point—off the brake and accelerator pedals. Your position will not be centered in the driver's seat but closer to the midline than usual because of leaving the injured right leg over the driveshaft hump. Tricky at first, but you and your left leg will soon adapt—and will be less dependent on others for the weeks or months ahead.

• • •Word to the Wise: SLIDING. Cloth-upholstered car seats are difficult to slide on; a square of heavy plastic, a garbage bag, or a piece of old vinyl tablecloth can make sliding less fatiguing.

Ready to bust out? Read on for added tips on traveling in the fast lane.

Driving Basics

Well, it's pretty certain that you never thought you'd be checking out how to enter and exit cars, but here goes.

Getting started: Approach the car door, and place your body far enough away so that on heaving the door open it doesn't hit you. Hold your strong-side crutch in the armpit grip in order to free up that hand—and give the door a *big yank*. For the armpit grip see Chapters 5 and 14.

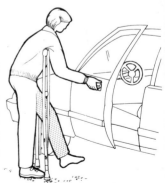

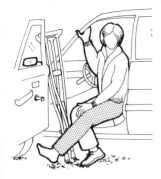

If you are still pretty weak or the door is very heavy, establish your crutches against the car, hold on to the car, and *then* yank.

Getting in: With the door open and the crutches back in their normal armpit position, hop forward to the seat. Take hold of the car *frame* with one hand, and get rid of the crutches—temporarily—by leaning them in the corner made where the door is hinged to the car. This efficient as well as foresighted move makes the crutches into a wedge—effectively hindering the doors of vehicles from developing minds of their own—and striking back at you.

> *Caution: Never* hold on to the car door itself unless it is wedged—since it is not stable.

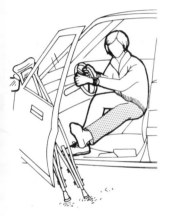

Sitting: Hands free, car tamed, and crutches established, sit down—that is, turn around, back up until your good leg is touching the seat, and, in general, follow the guidelines from Chapter 7.

• • • Word to the Wise: SEAT. The seat may need to be put back considerably, or you may need to scrunch yourself onto the center console in order to stuff yourself in—especially if you have a full-length leg cast.

Establishing the crutches: Bring the paired crutches into the car, and—between you and the door—place the tips on the car floor and the armpit heads between the corner of your seat back and the car frame, about where the shoulder seat belt is anchored. Just let them lie there.

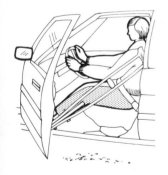

> *Note:* When crutches are paired on the door side in this fashion and you're the driver, they can be used as a foot rest for a left leg needing modest elevation. If you're a passenger, they can either be a prop in the center of the car or on the outer side, depending upon which leg needs raising.

• • • Word to the Wise: CRUTCH PLACEMENT. Whether you are the driver or the passenger, it is much more convenient and a major saver of energy to keep your crutches right next to you—rather than to toss them to or tug them from the back of your car. Your traveling companions will greatly appreciate the fact that you can stow and get them yourself, and you'll appreciate being able to make speedier getaways.

Getting out: O.K., you've arrived, time to get going. Stand the crutches in their "wedging-and-waiting" position at the angle of the vehicle door and vehicle frame, then get your body rotated outward and feet placed on the ground.

● ● ●Word to the Wise: TOTING. An important note for the saving of your time, energy, and sanity: if you have a purse or tote bag to lug with you, now's the moment to sling it over your shoulder (see Chapter 14) or to bring other paraphernalia within reach for easy retrieval once you are out of the car.

Getting up: Use your hands to push off from the car seat and to pull down on the door frame, grab your gear, grab your crutches, and it's off you go. Not bad, not bad.

Caution: If you use the car door for hoisting yourself, it *must* be wedged by your crutches.

Parking

Handicapped parking permit: It is truly a life-saver to have a permit that allows you reserved parking next to the entrances of office buildings, supermarkets, railroad stations, airline terminals, malls, and the like. With everything else you're putting up with, *do* take advantage of this right, which will keep you from getting discouraged about going places, which will help your independence, which will help days fly by. Even if your expected time on crutches may be only a few weeks, there will be many additional weeks of rehabilitation, when walking unnecessary distances will still be difficult. So whether it's crutches, cane, walker, or the pain and limp of an arthritic hip—find out how to "put yourself close."

Each municipality has its own regulations for temporary handicapped-parking permits, in addition to license plates for long-term mobility impairment. Generally, getting a permit requires that a form be signed by your doctor. Call your town or city government to find out how—*now!* You will discover that the luxury of those reserved spaces—so close to the action—will spoil you forever.

Checking the lay of the land: call ahead: It takes just a moment, so it's always a good idea to call ahead to places where parking might be a problem and find out the lay of the land. This is especially sensible for destinations where no reserved handicapped space is provided at all, and for those occasions when a lot of people are expected and you suspect you will end up in the back forty. In such cases, you may be allowed to park in certain areas normally prohibited to the general public. When attending large private receptions such as weddings, ask your host to save you a space at the front door or ask another guest to park your car for you.

Parking on hills: If you can avoid parking on hills, by all means do so. Control of the car doors is much harder on an incline, as is heaving yourself up from your seat. Getting your crutches positioned and ready to go isn't so easy either.

> *Note:* Avoidance of inclines is not only for those in which the *front end* of your car is pointing uphill but those in which *one side* of the car is markedly higher than the other.

AIRPLANE TRAVEL

Hampered as you are, you too can travel afar *and* on your own; it is much easier than you think. In fact you'll be amazed at times how many wheelchair travelers are lined up waiting for their flights at boarding gates—why shouldn't you, too? Full speed ahead for suggestions on how to take the trauma out of travel. See Chapter 19 for travel agencies specializing in travel for those who use mobility aids.

Airline Facilities

It is wise to call the individual airline that you are using to find out what assistance, services, and barriers will be present as you make your way from curbside at departure to ground transportation at your destination. Be specific as to what your situation is, and although you are probably only temporarily "un-able" or disabled, ask to speak to the person in charge of services for such travelers. When possible plan travel for off-peak hours and take direct flights. Above all, arrive early at the airport and leave extra time to make connecting flights.

Airline Seating

Bulkhead seat: If you are sporting a cast or have other problems requiring additional leg room, be sure to request a bulkhead seat. There is no guarantee that your travel agent or airline personnel can arrange this, but give them *plenty of advance notice* so they can try. Those accommodations get snapped up early.

Aisle seat: An aisle seat, with your injured limb closest to the aisle rather than on the inside, is another good choice for maximum comfort—and saves you from having to squeeze and scrunch by fellow passengers.

• • •Word to the Wise: CHECK-IN. Do not be timid. Even if you were unable to get the appropriate seat beforehand and are already at the check-in counter, hop up or wheel up and request accommodations more suitable to your situation. A bulkhead seat, at this stage, is probably out of the question, but gate attendants usually are happy to attempt an improvement of some sort. Lastly, once you are on the plane you may be able to switch seats with another traveler.

Large Luggage and Hand Luggage

Curbside check-in at your airline's departure area requires that you have your ticket in hand when you arrive—and by all means have it. Getting rid of your main luggage as soon as possible is essential for saving of energy and time.

On your landing, major metropolitan airports have sky caps to get your checked pieces to ground-transportation departure points—the extra expense of tipping should be anticipated. At smaller destinations, you will be dependent on good will and good nature.

For items that you carry with you on board: Simply stated—one piece of hand luggage is all that any person with limited mobility can manage when traveling by plane. In addition, since you will frequently be asking an airline attendant to carry your bag down an aisle or up the tricky stairs that smaller aircraft are equipped with, one such item is enough for you to keep track of or for someone else to have to carry.

Females: Make your hand luggage some type of smallish tote bag which can hold your reading matter *and* your purse, as well as any essentials such as medications, reading matter, a sweater, snack, or cosmetics—but nothing else that is not absolutely required. Taking a tote with interior compartments where you can isolate your wallet, ticket, keys, etc., often means you can dispense with the purse entirely.

Males and females: If possible, business papers should go into your single carry-all, as described above. If that's not feasible, let your briefcase be your single piece of hand luggage and fit everything else into it.

Caution: Be sure to pack essential medications in your carry-on bag in case your luggage gets lost or misdirected.

WHEELCHAIRS: THE WISE WAY TO GO

Granted that you may have logged countless miles on crutches or limped long distances with a cane, request—or have your travel agent request—a wheelchair at airport check-ins and at airplane disembarkations. Unless the airport is very, *very* small, do not get ambitious and attempt to hoof it yourself. Most airports are huge and spread out, and traversing them takes energy you should be saving.

In addition, no matter how careful you've been about the size of your hand luggage, even the smallest piece will make your trek through the terminal strenuous and laborious—again wasting valuable energy.

For your information and confidence enhancement, various aspects of wheelchair use within the airport facility are discussed.

Caution: Because of their congestion, airports are dangerous for individuals using mobility aids. Crowds of rushing people just do not notice that a person is slowed down by crutches or some other assistive device. Persons coming in from behind and darting in and out pose the most risk—because you can't see *them* to avoid collision, and they're too intent on weaving the fastest route between themselves and their destination to see *you*. Anyone traveling with you should walk just behind you—either pushing your wheelchair or blocking traffic if you're using crutches or a cane, or are dangerously slow or unsteady. If you are alone, the best tactic is to walk close to a wall whenever possible.

Wheelchair not present: If there's no chair waiting for you on arrival at the airport, don't panic. Inform the baggage or counter personnel, and one will come promptly.

Route to boarding gate: Your trip to the gate may take you through unfamiliar territory—back corridors, freight elevators, and the like—since the attendant cannot use escalators or stairs with a wheelchair.

Tipping: To show appreciation for the attendant's expertise and knowledge, a tip is usually offered for such service.

Wheelchair attendants: Wheelchair pushers—either friends, family, or travel personnel—often forget that footrests and an injured leg are not neat and tidy, but on the contrary stick out *beyond* the wheelchair—where they can be run into people, into doors, and into a lot of other things. So warn your pushers about those toes.

Establishing crutches and gear: Your hand luggage goes on your lap. Your crutches can be held upright by positioning the tips down on the wheelchair footrest next to the uninjured foot.

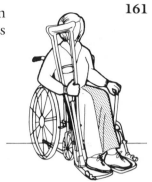

● ● ●Word to the Wise: REST ROOM NEEDS. Definitely use the airport rest room before boarding; plane facilities are notorious for limited room, not to mention the challenge of just getting to them. With the same goal in mind, go light on fluid intake before boarding and during the flight, as well.

Getting On and Off Airplanes by Wheelchair

At the boarding gate, major airports: Once you are pushed to the departure gate, check in with the airline personnel and get your seat assignment if you haven't already done so.

Then you and your chair will be parked nearby for "pre-boarding," when you and all passengers needing extra time will go on the plane ahead of other travelers. Your chair will be wheeled up (or down) the boarding ramp to the door of the plane, and there—if possible—you get up and use your crutches, cane, or walker, or get helped by an airline attendant.

Since airplane aisles are not only too narrow for wheelchairs but for most anything else as well, getting down them on crutches will probably require you to execute some fancy sideways sidling before—at last—you can settle in your seat. For help with sideways crutching, see Chapter 5.

> *Note:* Not able to walk at all? No problem. The airlines have a narrow-seated contraption on wheels, an "aisle chair," just for such situations—to which you are transferred. Be sure to alert airline personnel that you need such help when you make your reservations.

Boarding at small airports, flying in small planes: In these settings, it is quite possible that you and your wheelchair will be pushed out to where the plane is parked on the tarmac or be put onto a shuttle bus to get to your plane. (Such buses and planes generally have unusually difficult steps—more on those and buses in general below.)

Arrival at your seat: You've made it. You'll have to relegate your cherished crutches to an overhead storage area, or—in smaller

planes — they'll be stowed away by an airplane attendant for the duration of the flight.

● ● ●Word to the Wise: REMINDER. At this point, it is a good idea to
remind the attendant that you will need a wheelchair on landing.
Your destination airport will be informed by radio.

Nuthin' to do now but sit back and relax.

Arrival at your destination: Here's where you sit back and relax
a little bit more, while all your fellow passengers scurry and scuffle
madly in the stampede to disembark. You'll be last for obvious reasons,
and by the time you get to the door of the plane, a wheelchair will be
waiting. You will be taken wherever you wish to go, whether it is
baggage claim, the taxi stand, car-rental agency, or the waiting area at
the boarding gate for your connecting flight.

● ● ●Word to the Wise: MEETING SOMEONE. If you are being met,
arrange in advance of departure to join up at baggage claim. There
will be less risk of missing each other in case you are wheeled
through back by-ways on your journey to the luggage-retrieval
area. Additionally, the person who meets you will be able to help
carry your luggage when you're ready to leave.

Time to kill between flights: If you've time to squander, consider
going to an airport restaurant to relax over a snack and beverage — but
arrange with the wheelchair attendant in advance how and when you
will get a push back to the gate for your flight.

The Itty-Bitty Stairs of Itty-Bitty Planes

Sometimes you may ride planes that aren't all that small, but the stairs
up to them are small indeed — too narrow by far to use two crutches in
ascending the usual way. (Even if a cane or walker is your form of aid,
your leg strength may be inadequate for the steep grade.) How do you
cope?

Most basic: Well, one way is to choose the lowliest route —
meaning on your backside. It's guaranteed — and it's reassuringly safe —
but it's not too great for your traveling duds. Sometimes, though, it's
the only way — so traveling in "don't-care" clothes may be the answer.

Basic ascending: Standard stair techniques can be tried, of
course — in this case pairing both crutches under one arm and pulling
yourself up the stair railing or cable with the other (see Chapter 8).
Unfortunately, such cables are generally too low and slack to be much

help. That—along with the steep and exceptionally narrow stair treads such planes present—can make things pretty challenging and frequently impossible for normal non-weight-bearing crutch techniques.

"Pull me, push me":   Another alternative is to use your crutches to get onto the first stair—which is as far as *they* will be able to get. Then give them to an airline attendant—several such persons will be hovering anxiously nearby—and use the supporting railings, cables, or handgrips on both sides of the stair ramp to pull yourself up from one stair to the next while hopping as powerfully as you can on your working leg. This ascent can be quite dramatic because of all those attendant attendants—one of whom will be pulling you up from his or her position at the door of the plane and another of whom will be pushing you from behind.

Being carried: If it isn't ruled out due to your height and weight, don't eliminate this alternative in a case of desperate need.

Getting into smaller planes is definitely a "multiple-front" campaign, one worthy of a four-star general. Your dignified image—if you care anymore—will be a bit compromised by these methods, but whichever one you elect, the airline personnel will be 100 percent helpful and supportive (in some cases, literally). What they and your fellow travelers notice and respect are your grit and determination to get places. So, keep on trekkin'!

RIDING BUSES

The primary hurdle with buses is just that—the steps can be so high that they are hurdles indeed. Getting into one if you are using crutches may call all your strength and confidence into play. The dynamic strategy below will gain your entry into buses—promise—but don't skip review of the required crutch techniques in Chapter 8, in particular concerning stairs that are especially steep and "Advanced Ascending." "Advanced Descending" might be worth a peak also just to make sure you can get out with equal style at your destination. Then get on with the specific suggestions below.

> *Caution:* "Step hurdling"—if you're non-weight-bearing with crutches—is *advanced* stuff, for experts only. If in doubt about your strength and ability, corral a friend to "spot" you from behind, or use less advanced stair-management techniques, not forgetting the option of the basic "bottom boogie."

Push off: From the tripod position explode *extra* hard with your arms and crutches, and *heave* your good foot up onto that high-rising tread. Here's where a buddy can be behind you for safety's sake as well as to provide a push if required. Once your foot's placed, take a quick moment to regroup, or forge right on ahead — your choice.

"Your choice" means no law says you *have* to rush here. When your foot has landed, you can leave the crutches planted behind you until ready to push on. The knee of that good leg — placed up so high — will of course be in a *very* flexed position, and your weight will be hanging out behind you — supported by the planted crutches.

Monumental push-off number two: Here's where you astound the other riders with an *impressive* crutch "push-off," bringing those sticks up to the stair, while simultaneously and powerfully straightening the leg planted on the stair.

Ascending: Once you have hoisted yourself onto the bottom step, you can ascend the remaining steps using Basic Technique — both crutches under the strong-side armpit and using the railing for help — or using Advanced Technique — crutches on either side.

Descending: Leaving the bus will also be a choice between Basic and Advanced techniques, depending upon your strength and skill.

Take your time, take a friend — but take a ride.

RIDING TRAINS

Train travel has become a lot more accessible than it used to be, making it a good choice for a person with mobility problems. Federal laws have caused revamping of the major stations, making elevators accessible and entrances into railroad cars level with station platforms. On Amtrak, employees get special training in traveler assistance, and meals can be requested to be brought to your seat if walking or crutching in a moving train is too hazardous. For more on Amtrak, see Chapter 19.

BOATS, HANG GLIDERS, DOG SLEDS, AND OTHER EXOTIC VEHICLES

If your fondest desire includes boating or some other seemingly impossible feat, do not give up on it. By now — with all the techniques you've mastered, plus a dab or two of advance planning, ingenuity, and innovation — you may have adapted enough to be able to participate in your favorite activity. Failing that, go spectate instead.

Boats: When the tide's out a ramp to your boat can look steeper than Mount Everest. Intimidating, to be sure, but don't let it keep you from your craft. Go Very Basic (on your backside) or just plain Basic (both crutches on one side and using the railing on the other). If the tide's still out on your return, choose your preferred ascending method — and get someone to give you boosts on the behind. For review of stair techniques see Chapter 8.

Getting into or onto a boat from a dock may require sitting on the dock or a piling and swinging yourself over to the boat on your posterior. Not too elegant, but better that you try — and get in place for some fun. And that goes for recreation in general: try — and get in place for some fun.

Ships: If you had a great vacation planned and had to give it up because of an injured leg, substituting a cruise is a wonderful option. Many ships have been adapted with the mobility challenged in mind, which — at the moment — means you, too. See Chapter 19 for relevant information.

PACKING AND UNPACKING

Luggage: Once at your destination, however you got there, you'll find life a lot easier to manage if your clothes are in flat, firm-sided, traditional suitcases. The duffle-type makes it very hard to find your clothes and is harder to get in and out of in general.

Arrangement of clothes: Another reason for the traditional suitcase is that you will want to keep your clothes in it rather than putting them away. Getting clothes into drawers takes energy, and getting drawers opened and shut takes energy. Leaving clothes where they are does not take energy. Even more energy will be saved when it is time to leave — because the clothes have never been unpacked.

Placement of suitcase: Wherever you are staying, you're in luck if your room has a spare bed. Place your suitcase right there. A bed is a good height for you to work from, and it affords extra space on which to neatly lay your clothes. If you absolutely must get rid of your suitcase, let the clothes all be on the bed. If there is no spare bed, use the top of a bureau, desk, or table — either for the suitcase or neat piles of clothing.

Getting comfortable on the road: Only you know what you need. If it's extra pillows for leg elevation, a chair for the bathroom or stair landing, water at the bedside, or whatever, make arrangements with the lodging management or your host.

Portable weights for rehabilitative exercise: Who are you conning to carry the heavy cuff or cast-iron doughnut weights required to bring your quadriceps back to fightin' form? Car travel and iron for pumping is one thing, but taking weights on trains or into the friendly skies is another. Not to worry, a solution has been found. Someone smart has come up with vinyl cuffs that you fill with water when you've settled in at your destination. The cuffs are calibrated to equate water levels with exact amounts of weight. They aren't as easy to use as real weights, but with them there's no need to stay home to work the laggard leg; you can travel guilt free, *plus* keep your recovery on track. See Chapter 19 for obtaining travel cuffs.

Handicapped parking permit: If you're planning to drive at your destination, be sure to take your permit with you.

DESTINATIONS

You may never have had time to go to museums or zoos, see movies or plays, shop, or just goof off. How about getting in a few wild and woolly wanderings now that injury has put time on your hands? *Don't* just catch up on long-avoided home projects. Create diversions for yourself. See below for practical hints on cultural and shopping adventures.

● ● ●Word to the Wise: CHECK AHEAD. The key to attendance at concerts, theaters, sporting events, etc., is checking out accessibility in advance.

What is accessibility? Accessibility is the arrangement of architectural and transportation details in such a way as to give people in wheelchairs or using crutches and other aids the opportunity to enter, leave, and get around buildings, to circulate in urban or suburban areas, and to participate at recreational facilities of all kinds. This includes the presence or lack of curb-cuts, handicapped parking, elevators, appropriate entry doors and rest rooms, and wheelchairs available in museums—to name just a few. *Check ahead!*

National Parks

Getting around in one of our wonderful parks may seem out of the question when a painful patella or fractured fibula is dragging you down. Help is at hand with *Access America: An Atlas and Guide to the National Parks for Visitors with Disabilities*. For details on this exceptional book, see Chapter 19.

Museums, Zoos

Museums and zoos are like airports—the only sensible way to traverse the hard floors and long paths and view the displays without being felled by fatigue or foot failure is by wheelchair. Use the freight and exhibit elevators to get from one level to another.

• • •Word to the Wise: WHEELCHAIRS. Most museums have wheelchairs, but call ahead to make sure. Go with a pal. The pal can push you as well as share the pleasure. Ditto for zoos—although unfortunately you'll probably have to bring your own wheelchair.

Theaters, Stadiums

Theaters and stadiums can be challenging because of crowds and stairs. Always call ahead, have a friend stop by the box office, or write in your ticket requests—in order to explain your situation and get appropriate seating. A leg cast *requires* an aisle seat, and even if your limb has been liberated, its restricted range of motion and your comfort make aisle seating mandatory. If you have to go up stairs, have someone "spot" you from behind when both ascending and descending. Since a wheelchair is now routinely accommodated in many new theaters and stadiums, you no longer have to miss the hottest musical, the Super Bowl, or the Indy 500.

Malls, Department Stores, Restaurants, Public Buildings

Accessibility: Such buildings are often furnished with highly visible escalators and revolving doors—equipment not exactly guaranteed to raise the spirits of anyone with a broken ankle or ligament repair. Read on for reassurances.

Elevators: Elevators seem frequently to be non-existent. Do not be put off, do not stay home. Elevators do exist—at the very least for the freight—and you, along with moms and kiddies in strollers, will be allowed aboard.

• • •Word to the Wise: CHECK AHEAD. Call ahead to find out where elevators are located, where the store entrance closest to the elevator is located, and if there is parking nearby. Save your valuable energy for some heavy-duty shopping, or whatever other amusement you're contemplating.

Revolving doors: Revolving doors are generally flanked by heavy swinging doors that can be pushed or pulled.

> *Caution:* If there are no doors of the latter type, wait until you can enter the revolving door alone—with a friend or passerby guarding the approaches so nobody comes in behind and whirls you off your feet. See Chapter 9 for more tips on safe use of revolving doors.

Excessive shopping: The solution to overenthusiastic shopping or bulky, heavy packages is to request the help of a stock boy to carry them to the car for you.

Let your fingers do the walking: With smaller or local stores, you may be able to save your energy by asking that they bring your telephoned order out to you in your car. If opening heavy doors is not your strong suit—even after reading Chapter 9—alert the store of your expected arrival so they can help you.

Buying clothes: Trying on clothes is exhausting even if both your legs are perfect. Take your purchases home and try them on there or buy from mail-order catalogues.

Eating out: Many restaurants now advertise their accessibility, so even if you need a wheelchair to get out and about, you should be able to enjoy someone else's cooking and clean-up. Be sure to phone ahead, however, to verify that the restaurant's concept of accessibility means no stairs in entering or in reaching the rest room.

KEEPING OPTIONS OPEN

Summertime gardening: All is not totally lost just because of a mashed metatarsus or a gnashed knee. If grubbing in dirt is your delight, become a container cultivator: substitute seat-height horticulture for kneeling and bending in the earthy plot you love so well.

Possibilities are earthenware pots, redwood planters, cut-off wine barrels, or anything lying around that will hold soil and let water run out. Have them placed up on blocks at the correct height and reap crops of herbs, lettuce, tomatoes, and the like right at your doorstep—and worry no longer that rabbits, raccoons, or other pests will eat them out from under your nose.

Wintertime gardening, bird watching, brain exercise, and innovation: Cold weather, ice, and snow will prevent anyone hobbling and wobbling from doing most of their favorite outdoor activities. To keep fingernails dirty and split for the summer season to come, consider terrarium gardening, a challenging and rewarding form of indoor container horticulture.

Birds can brighten up a window and the winter scene immensely if you put out a feeder and suet; a bird book and a pair of binoculars will increase your pleasure. A tank full of colorful fish does the same thing, and cleaning modern tanks is no longer a laborious chore. Pets of many kinds—from kittens to gerbils to canaries—are great antidotes for long days of enforced inactivity.

Exercise your gray cells by taking advantage of community or school-sponsored courses that you may never have had time for previously.

Or there's innovation—a combination of interest and ingenuity—which you can employ to find your own ways to use days of recovery wisely and wonderfully.

Figuring out how you can participate in your favorite activities—either partially or as a spectator—can become a goal in itself. Meeting that challenge—solving it and doing something that seemed impossible—can become a reward in itself.

By now you know you can get to a lot of places that may have seemed out of the question when your injury or operation first occurred. With all the skills and techniques you've acquired, and the innovative, ingenious frame of mind going with them, you should be able to manage or improvise in many types of situations that no one, you or anybody else, could have imagined. Here's hoping you are doing just that.

16   Caring for Kids When You Can Hardly Walk

It's time to roll out and rev up your stores of untapped imagination and innovation if you are on crutches or in some other restrictive stage of recovery and have a baby or young children to take care of. Because of the enormous variation in age, activity levels, motor abilities, and levels of concentration, there is no one strategy that will work for all children or all age groups.

Some of the ideas here may fit your situation perfectly, others may have to be adapted, and still others you will have to invent spontaneously. Most situations will not be identical. Use your smarts, be flexible, keep a sense of humor—and this too shall pass.

GENERAL GUIDELINES

Use of a wheelchair: If you are restricted to crutches, tire easily, or have a horribly heavy cast to heave around, utilizing a wheelchair part-time will make caring for a child infinitely more manageable and infinitely less tiring. See below for suggestions tailored separately for infants and toddlers, as well as Chapter 6.

Conservation of energy: This is an important consideration for anyone trying to care for him or herself as well as for children. Preplan and try to establish consistent routines with the goal in mind of saving your strength. Using a wheelchair temporarily will be a big help in this department.

Require the children to rest in some way or other—either napping or playing on their beds—and be sure to rest yourself at the same time. Using crutches or other aids, or walking with a limp, takes a lot out of you.

Flexible attitude: If necessary, bend the rules and let things slide a bit during your recovery.

Accessibility of child: Young children—or any child that cannot be totally trusted to act prudently whether alone or with others — must be accessible (within reach or close calling distance) at all times.

This may mean rather drastic restructuring of your child's freedom. Depending on age, he or she may need to be prevented from entering rooms where you are unable to supervise — for this, doors can be shut or baby gates installed.

For a while your child may become an "indoors child" — playing exclusively in the house if you cannot get outdoors. Even if you can get out to your yard or sidewalk, there remains the responsibility of being physically able to rescue and remove your child should an accident occur. Although fresh air is nice for children, it is not mandatory, especially if proper supervision or "rescue-ability" is impossible.

Organization: As with all other facets of your life right now, you can save yourself time and future problems by selection, elimination, and organization of chores and activities. Routines for your children are also very important during this period, to counteract the natural tendency to want "to do their own thing." See Chapter 2 for more suggestions on organization.

Playing with your children: Depending upon your own situation, your bed is the perfect spot to play with younger children. However, as your recovery progresses and once you've learned how to get down to the floor and back up again (see Chapter 7), there'll be things you can do there better than on a bed, like rolling over with your child, roughhousing (maybe), finger painting, or playing with cars and trucks.

Safety: You will have to be *much* more careful about all safety hazards, since you are not able to react as quickly to a fall or some object falling on your child. Caution family members not to leave *anything* around in the kitchen, bathrooms, or anywhere that might harm a young child — after having first toddler-proofed the house to the best of your ability.

Start slow: Keep things nice and simple until you learn the ropes of coping with kids when you've a broken leg or casted ankle. Get the little ones accustomed to the "new but temporary you" *inside* your home before venturing beyond.

Accept help: It goes without saying that you will avail yourself of any help that is responsible and suitable for your child or children. Ask, however, that when the children are returned to your care — either from outdoors or from somewhere else in your home — that they not be in an overexcited state, which will only make your job harder. Suggest a 5- to 10-minute "cool down" before return — having a story read or playing a quiet game.

CARE OF AN INFANT

Safety of the Infant

Of prime importance, the methods normally used for their protection will not be substantially altered despite your lack of mobility. You'll just be more careful that all customary procedures are followed. If a baby is beginning to crawl or stand, a harness can be temporarily employed.

Equipment for the Care of Babies

Use of a wheelchair: Getting your baby moved from room to room is a cinch with a wheelchair. Your lap is ready and waiting for everything from feeding to changing. Armrest trays are available for wheelchairs, or a soft pillow — placed on your lap — can cradle the baby. Putting the baby into a "front pack" or Snugli will leave both your hands free for other tasks. When you resume walking, the infant (or toddler) can take your place in the wheelchair. As you push it, the child will be entertained and transported — while at the same time you will be strengthening your leg and practicing walking skills.

The crib: A portable crib is highly recommended for any immobilized parent trying to take care of a baby. Portable cribs are narrow enough to go through most doors, and in a single-floor home wherever you go the baby can go with you — to play as well as sleep in the crib. If you have stairs in your home, someone else will have to bring down the baby and crib in the morning and return them at bedtime.

When your infant is able to stand, the mattress of any type of crib is usually lowered. However, that now makes care of the child much more difficult — particularly if you are fairly immobile. Consider temporarily keeping the mattress at the higher level — or returning it there — and using a harness that permits the child to sit but not stand.

Umbrella stroller: Such strollers are easily portable and are another method of getting the baby around as well as providing a place to sleep and play. As these strollers are extremely lightweight, you should be able to move one even if you're on crutches. See Chapter 14 for relevant techniques. The baby can be put right next to wherever you've settled yourself for either feeding or entertaining. If you have trouble getting down to the stroller level, seat yourself first before transferring the baby in or out.

A is for Apron: Caring for an infant means bottles, powders, creams, and the like. Your apron is indispensable here (see Chapter 14).

C is for Chair: Another option, both for diapering the infant and for any other care given at cribside, is the bar-height chair or stool recommended for use in the kitchen (see Chapter 13). Perch or sit as your situation allows, establish your crutches — if used — to either side, and tend the little one.

Playpen: If you are non-weight-bearing or have a full-length cast, a portable playpen is useful only if someone is available to lift the baby in and out.

Infant seat: Infant seats are generally adjustable, flat for sleeping and tilted for feeding and playing. Since the baby can sleep, eat, and play all in one place — and right at your side — you save energy, and the baby is both supervised and safe.

Front packs, Snuglies: These papooselike sacks for carrying infants on the chest place the weight — as does the all-purpose apron — solidly in the center where your balance will be least compromised. If you have good stability and are strong enough for the infant's extra weight — and the babe is not a jumping jack — this might be an option for a person using crutches or other aids. Try it out at home first.

> *Caution:* You should get your doctor's permission before using a front pack for your child.

Baby walkers: If your injury allows you to lower a prewalking child into a walker, hours of active fun are possible. Sitting yourself down first and then putting the child into the walker is one method of getting him or her settled. As children approach the walking stage, however, they can move very fast in these wheeled contraptions, and inappropriate rooms — and, above all, stairs — must be blocked off.

Techniques for the Care of Babies

In caring for your baby the most important consideration is immediate and easy accessibility.

Reaching baby: A "draw" sheet underneath can be used to pull the baby closer so your balance is not compromised. The draw sheet can be a folded-up sheet or a changing pad.

Reaching objects in the crib or on the floor around the crib: The use of any type of reacher, such as barbecue tongs, will help your safety and your sanity. If it's feasible, you can tie toys to crib bars with soft shoe laces or strips of rag.

Diapering: Although you may have always stood to diaper your baby, this is certainly a routine you might want to change. Sitting down is safest, and your own bed—suitably protected—is a good place for both you and the baby. The crib should be placed adjacent so the baby can be safely transferred, a receptacle for the diapers should be handy, and cleaning supplies can be on a large lazy susan in easy reach or in a lightweight plastic basket (see Chapter 14). Have toys available wherever you diaper to keep the process from becoming an unpleasant struggle.

Breast feeding: Needless to say, you can still breast feed your baby even if an accident has thrown your leg into a cast and you into a tailspin. You'll find it easier, though, if you place a pillow or two onto your lap to raise the baby to a comfortable height as well as to cushion the cast. If the baby's crib is right next to your bed and if you're using your bed as baby's entertainment center during your recovery, breast feeding should be relatively simple, since no walking is involved.

Bottle feeding: Bottle feeding is more complicated because the milk doesn't just come out of the "faucet" as it does in breast feeding. However, with all the strategies of fetching and carrying you've been introduced to, it's doubtful that you will have problems getting the bottle and solid food to your baby. If it is a bottle your baby is getting, he or she doesn't have to be on your lap, of course—an infant seat that can be rocked is a good spot both for an easily induced nap after feeding and for general soothing, as well as for keeping the child in one accessible place.

Keeping a bottle cold and handy for nighttime feedings can be accomplished by using a small picnic cooler or wide-mouthed picnic jug filled with ice. Food for both you and the baby can be kept this way for daytime ease, if you are going to be left on your own and have difficulty getting to or using the kitchen.

Bathing: The easiest place to bathe an infant is your kitchen sink. It is both higher and generally larger than a bathroom sink, probably has a handy spray hose, and affords space to lay a towel for drying the baby. If you have an infant seat that is not covered in fabric, it can be placed right into the sink, making bathing even safer and easier since there will be no chance of the baby's slipping from your grasp. Bring the portable crib or stroller right alongside the sink so there is minimal transfer distance. Your bar stool or chair should be available for your use.

A plastic tub placed onto a table of convenient height or onto your bed is another way to bathe the baby, but getting water to the tub may be a problem if you are using crutches. However, if you can get someone to do the water toting, it does allow you to perform this enjoyable task. Disposable "chucks," available at medical-supply stores, are an efficient way to protect the bed, and a tub small enough to get between your spread legs will be easiest for handling of the infant.

CARE OF TODDLERS AND YOUNG CHILDREN

Safety of the child: This is of prime importance, and you will have to adapt both your house and your ways. Be willing to install portable baby gates across doors and stairs, close or lock doors, put away breakables, lock up cleaning supplies, eliminate inappropriate fans, cover electrical outlets, and use a harness. You are *not* denying your children—you are protecting and keeping them from harm until normalcy returns.

In general, keeping children busy keeps them out of trouble.

● ● ●Word to the Wise: CHILDPROOFING. If doors or cupboards have no built-in locks, hooks and eyes can be temporarily attached instead.

 If the child is in your sole care at nighttime, make sure that everything that might harm the child is put away. There will be less likelihood of injury should the little one wake and get going before you do in the morning. Depending upon age, tamper-proof gates will restrict the child to its room, and a harness will restrict it to bed. Balance that, however, against the need of a child to get to you if he's ill or having bad dreams.

 If there is any hazard for children in touching or playing with your assistive equipment, be sure your children are made aware of it. Walkers can be tippy to pull down on or hold on to, and the wheels of a moving wheelchair can catch fingers. In general, it is certainly best for youngsters not to touch, play with, or use your equipment in any way except in conjunction with your own use.

Discipline: This is a difficult area, but the advantage with the toddler and young-child set is that privileges and treats can be denied if they fail to cooperate. A blend of withholding when justified, relaxation of some requirements, and consistency on your part—as well as flexibility and humor—will help. It's a real balancing act.

 However, if you say "no," make sure you can stop the child from doing what you have forbidden, and never threaten to punish unless you can follow through. This may allow some unpleasant behavior to get by—but it also underlines that when you say something you mean it, which will improve obedience in the future. A harness can be a practical solution for the very mischievous child who is unable to cooperate.

Emphasize the importance of coming when called and other requirements related to safety and managing the home; the children must feel and understand the necessity. Demonstrate by concrete action that they will miss out on something fun by not coming; if necessary a spank can be used for emphasis.

Most displeasure, however, should be verbal and focus only on the action that was done or not done by the child. Avoid demeaning or attributing unpleasant character traits to a child in the heat of anger. Try to finish off any necessary discipline with a hug; after all, you want them to cooperate or come to you, not antagonize or avoid you.

Independence of the young child: Children can do a lot for themselves but need extra time in the doing. Allow and allot extra time, and your crutch *dependence* may produce *independent* offspring. They will also learn at an early age that they can be a tremendous help.

Explain to them any equipment you use, why you are using it, and how they can aid you in using it. Instruct them how to safely get down off of beds and chairs.

Imitation: Two- to three-year-olds may try to imitate your disability — limping badly or wanting to have a cast just like yours. This is harmless and natural, and will soon pass if ignored. Otherwise you can turn the interest to your advantage by creating play situations using items in the home to substitute for the real thing: a little leg can be "casted" with rags, sturdy sticks can be make-believe crutches and canes, you and the little one can alternate playing doctor and patient — the possibilities are many.

Equipment for Care of Toddlers and Young Children

In addition to the suggestions for babies, the following may prove helpful:

Using a wheelchair: Most children find it fun to get up onto a lap and be wheeled around — a ride is a treat for them — which makes their cooperation easier to achieve. And for you, scooting in a wheelchair after a toddler is more efficient than chasing on crutches. Once there you can scoop the little kid up, scold properly if necessary, and then hug warmly, whereas on crutches it's a complicated campaign of establishing yourself, then establishing your crutches — while the little rascal escapes.

Small children also like to stand or sit on wheelchair foot rests for rides. It's a cozy spot to hold on to a parent's legs while drinking a bottle, playing, or just looking up at mom or dad.

Harness: A harness sounds cruel, but it can provide safety — as well as controlled freedom for your child—that may be impossible to achieve any other way. Luckily, children are very adaptable, particularly if you, yourself, do not waver in requiring harnesss use. Attach the harness by its straps to the leg of your chair or bed or any solid, immovable object. Increase the roaming range of the child—if you like—by lengthening the ties in some fashion.

If you have a suitable play area outside a door yet do not want to be out yourself, screw in a large eye screw and attach the harness. The little one will enjoy being "reeled in like a fishie" when play time is up.

You may want to use a harness in your toddler's crib also, particularly if there is a chance of the child's falling out. The harness can be adjusted so that the tyke can sit and play but not stand and fall.

Techniques for Care of Toddlers and Young Children

Bathing: A toddler is generally able to get in and out of a tub, so your main role will be supervision. A good place for this might be your own bathroom, where you have the chair that allows you to rest (see Chapter 10)—as well as to get lower and closer to the child. A chair or stool can also be put in the child's bathroom.

Feeding: If your children are old enough, the fridge can have bottles and food placed on a lower shelf where they can help themselves. A low footstool may help in reaching the door pull.

Play activities: Innovation is imperative if the child's normal activities are no longer possible due to your injury—but your injury may also be an opportunity to do things with your child that you have been unable to do before. A blackboard is especially handy because letters or drawings can be erased and improved easily, and there's less chance of the damage to bedcovers, rugs, or walls that paint or crayons can cause. Storytelling is fun when either you or the child starts the story and the other one finishes it. Building blocks—from Lego plastic to old-fashioned wooden—are great passers of time if an adult is involved to keep the buildings growing and varied.

MANAGING THE OLDER CHILD

Older children have school, can largely take care of themselves, and probably already have well-ingrained habits; nevertheless much of the advice aimed at younger children will prove equally sensible for the older ones. Most of the difference will be a result of attitude: the small child wants to please, the older one doesn't find that so important anymore.

Older children may be embarrassed by your disability, even though it's temporary. Your using a wheelchair or walker—even crutches—makes *them* stand out, something most adolescents abhor. Frequently your problems will be ignored or avoided entirely. Their coping mechanisms have not yet had sufficient experience with injury or illness.

Strategies for Coping with Older Children

"Being there":   You won't be able to carpool your child to a Saturday swim meet or take him or her to get the latest in athletic footwear as easily as before your accident or operation, so take this time to listen better—*listen, not talk.* Although you may be in your most vibrant thirties or forties, your adolescent equates you to a centenarian and relegates your valuable parental experiences to the remotest times of predinosaur history. Just be there.

Enlist aid: Some help should be given gratis, but since most teenagers run through allowances as if the money were only meant to last a day in the first place, paying them fixed fees for chores that you cannot do is reasonable and persuasive. It is best not to pay in advance or be conned into paying in advance. Pay on completion of the task, making sure it is done to *your* satisfaction, not the youngster's. You are the one paying.

You would not have chosen knee reconstruction or foot surgery as a way of getting to know your children better but, like it or not, you will. And that can't be all bad.

Family and Friends: What You Can Do to Help

17

"Being there" for your incapacitated relative or friend—by visiting, providing emotional support, doing errands, or actual physical assistance—is really needed at this time. Without a doubt he or she is reeling from the shockwaves that extended immobility imparts. Even if one is dealing with scheduled surgery, it can be hard to imagine beforehand just how difficult it is to do all of life's little chores—getting one's clothes out of drawers and closets, making breakfast, feeding the dog, entering a car, or opening the door at work. Support and understanding definitely make it easier.

However, sometimes it is assumed by the provider that help of whatever kind is "best" for their relative or friend, with little consideration of individual sensibilities. Sometimes the underlying attitude is that after all, they're lucky to get *any* help. The suggestions offered here may or may not fit the particular situation or cirumstances with which you are coping, but they will provide ideas and perspectives.

Avoid being judgmental. What may appear an insignificant or trivial physical restriction to you can be monumental for other people. Many reactions and perceptions will depend upon age, physical fitness, amount of mobility lost, and amount of time needed to recover. A lot will also depend upon what the individuals involved were planning to do with their time in the near and maybe not-so-near future. Perhaps they were going on vacation, were about to participate in a special tournament or athletic endeavor—or training for one; perhaps they are *indispensable* at home or on the job, or simply *can't* miss work, a meeting, or deadline. A "simple" sprained ankle—and a sprain only sounds simple—can wreck all sorts of plans, obligations, and aspirations. An accident—by the nature of its being—is never convenient; even a scheduled operation is rarely convenient.

Friends are in a special category. They *choose* to connect with their buddy, their office associate, their work-crew companion, or their

179

teammate — families are generally involved willy-nilly. Both are needed. Don't fall into the category that Dimitri Bilozerchev, the "czar" of Russian gymnasts, spoke about after his leg was shattered in a car accident: "Finally you realize who are your true friends, and who are not. That is a fact you realize when something serious happens. I got rid of all my naiveté, all my illusions." If you're a friend, or even just an acquaintance, read on to see how you can fit in and how best to go about it.

Independence

It is easy to confuse "doing for" with "caring about." At times family and friends unwittingly limit or prevent achievable independence. Resist the "feeling good to be needed" trap and the similar one of "doing for someone" when you're really doing it *for you* — because it's easier for you. Although it may take restraint as well as more effort, you *can* show you care without necessarily doing everything for a person — and in the long run it's much, much better for that person. Said another way by a homespun philosopher: "We ought to be careful not to do for a fellow what we only intended to help him do."

Mobility aids — crutches, canes, walkers, and wheelchairs — make independence possible. Sometimes individuals resist using a particular device because of their dislike of drawing attention to themselves or because of their fear of becoming dependent on the aid. Help your friend or relative to realize that mobility aids are *liberating* — not confining — and that using them as needed will speed the rejoining of life's mainstream.

Ability to Choose

Another aspect of independence to be respected is freedom of choice. In "sparing" one's wife, one's husband, or one's parent the opportunity to make needed decisions, you are performing no favor. On the contrary, frequently it is to spare *oneself* the trouble of getting the choice made or the consequences of the choice once made. Being limited by what one can do should not limit one's freedom to choose.

Regaining Strength

It helps to remember, also, that when you perform the activity you ought only to help with, *you* become stronger; your recovering friend or family member gets stronger when *he* or *she* does it — as well as getting a useful ego boost in the department of self-reliance.

Don't hold back from taking the first step to offer sympathy and help to someone who's had an accident or an operation just because you don't know them very well. They will be even more touched by your concern—so follow your instincts.

Only offer to help if you are willing to carry through and—more important—have the time and opportunity to do so.

Avoid making "open-ended offers" of help—"call-me-if-you-need-me" offers that leave the burden of asking on the person who needs it. Try to be specific about what you can do or what day or evening you are free to fill in or do chores that your relative or friend can't. If he or she is uncertain about what these might be, ask permission to check with persons closer to the situation who might know.

Another way to contribute is to do chores or errands for those helpers who are more involved in physical care or actually at the hospital—rather than being just one more of many visitors who tire the patient. This can be continued after your friend or relative is doing better—to allow time off for others.

Do not cancel unless absolutely necessary.

Be sensitive to the fact that some people's sense of worth and self-esteem—power, even—is tied up in being able to do everything for themselves or in directing others to do those things. Sometimes adjustments to situations of helplessness can result in authoritarian behavior to mask real feelings underneath. If such is the case, yet aid is needed, try to provide it—if appropriate—when the individual is otherwise occupied.

Offering Help: Physical Assistance

Most people are ill at ease with persons who are injured or suffering. They're afraid they'll say the wrong thing, appear too intrusive, or assist clumsily and improperly. Yet knowing the struggle their relative or buddy is making to do the simplest task makes them want to make it easier. The best solution is to ask matter-of-factly if assistance is needed—"May I help you? or "Would a helping hand be of any use?"—and let the individual tell you what and when.

Be sure also to find out *how*. If it's help standing that's needed, have your friend or relative explain precisely what you are to do. If it's help getting out of bed, understand clearly what he or she will be doing and what you will be doing. (Later on in this chapter you will find suggested techniques that can be used in providing safe and efficient physical assistance.)

Be alert. Don't offer assistance only at the moment when the relative or friend has finally managed: notice instead the first intimations of struggle, and offer then.

Remember, you're on a tightrope — balancing your assistance with the need to respect an individual's independence as well as with the necessity of his doing things for himself to further strength and recovery. Generally speaking, assistance with basic physical actions will become less and less of a factor as recovery progresses.

What to Ask

It's not taboo to ask about your friend's health or how he or she is feeling. It's a normal part of "family-ship" and friendship, and never to ask would indicate you didn't care. Be sure to "invite" a truthful response, though — one that will let your friend unwind — and skip any "keep the chin up" moralizing.

On the other hand, don't be too inquisitive about details: a person's privacy should be respected. Concepts of privacy differ, but if you're sensitive you'll be able to tell when you're invading someone's "space." If privacy turns out not to be a factor, you'll probably get more details than you really want to hear, anyway — which is where being a friend and good listener comes in.

What to Do

Listen. Hear. Your friend or relative may be in pain. Everything will be colored by that, and he or she will need a comforting hand and an understanding ear. If the pain factor is negligible, frustration is certainly present. Frequently anger is, too, particularly if an accident was someone else's fault.

Dr. Bernie Siegel writes in *Love, Medicine and Miracles* that his own son told him — at such a time — that "I don't need answers, I need someone to listen." Listening is the highest form of caring.

The support of caring families and friends can help the severely injured accept their condition — which may include the loss of former prowess and skills. The tightrope to be walked teeters between being caring but not intrusive, being ready and willing to help without taking over.

And always, being ready to listen.

Respond to frustration and worry without comment on what the future will bring. Do not minimize: acknowledge fears, give them validity. Sometimes the best thing is to hold a hand and simply say, "I'm so sorry."

If there are concrete signs of improvement, appropriate notice of them can be made. Expect, however, to have improvement put down or belittled; frustration, anger, and dismay at what still has to be achieved are uppermost for the patient.

If your advice is asked—perhaps you've had similar surgery or have experience in some field which would be of aid to your friend or relative—give it in such a way that it can be freely rejected.

What Not to Say

Well-meaning friends and relatives invariably project unrelenting optimism—that all is "hunky-dory" even if their friend will be in a cast for months, unable to work, and has no insurance. The catastrophe—and such it is for most people suddenly immobilized for whatever reason—is, in effect, not allowed to exist. Most often it is denied through constant hymns to a rosy future—despite the fact that the future may well include decidedly unrosy restrictions on activities once taken for granted and pastimes that are particularly cherished.

Ritualized remarks—such as "I know how you must feel"—often have the effect of implying the friend's situation is familiar and commonplace. On the contrary, unless you have been through the very same ordeal yourself, you probably have little or no idea how your friend or relative is feeling; one hopes that what they are going through is not familiar or commonplace for anyone.

Avoid talking about yourself—particularly during the immediate aftermath of an accident, an injury, or an operation. Above all, don't compare the patient's situation to something similar in your life. Your friend needs an ear—not a mouth.

Ritualized questioning—"How are you?"—frequently makes ill or injured persons uncomfortable, particularly if they are on a long, long "road back." They know most people are not interested in an honest answer about the pains, the setbacks, or the small advances that may have occurred since they last talked. If you do ask the question, be ready to listen and to allow the person to say that things aren't great. If skipping the ritual "How are you?" question seems in order, just say, "I've been thinking of you," and go on with your news or business from there.

Ritualized cheerfulness — "It will be over before you know it" and similar platitudes — insinuates exaggeration of symptoms on the part of individuals, implying, even, that they're feeling sorry for themselves. Belittling the difficulties of the situation only makes it harder to accept loss of independence and mobility. Better to say, "What an ordeal you're going through." Be careful also with that old standby, "You must be feeling better — you look better." Appearances are often deceptive.

Ritualized dishonesty — of the sort that says that everything is fine when it clearly isn't — should be avoided. Fall back on being a good listener, and leave forecasts about the future to medical personnel.

Advice or criticism — or anything smacking of it — is always going to be taken better if it comes from someone in a white coat.

Pronouncements of a philosophical nature are usually resented, as they suggest a wisdom on the part of the visitor that the patient does not have. And when something drastic has happened — say a bad auto accident with your friend's car crushed and his leg too — he's not ready for such insights anyway.

Ritualized optimism, philosophy, cheerfulness — all make the visitor feel good, but the anguish (which may or may not be expressed) of the injured friend or relative is often glossed over, put down, brushed aside, or ignored.

Isolation Imposed

If all friends and family insist that "he's getting better," proclaim "isn't she lucky it wasn't worse?" and predict that "he'll be out and about in no time," the patient often feels isolated. No matter what truth there is in those reflections — truths he undoubtedly knows for himself — his innermost thoughts are probably quite different. He or she also may feel, because of the contemporary emphasis on being macho and strong and brave no matter what, that it is unseemly to admit to problems or pain. If he's forced to maintain a "good front," isolation may be imposed.

Besides emotional isolation, there's the obvious isolating separation due to inability to participate physically in former activities. Some individuals reach out on their own to friends from work or recreation; others may need you to make the first overture.

Families should pay particular attention to including their parent, child, sibling, husband, wife, or other relative in every decision possible. Just because they are off their feet doesn't mean they've "lost their marbles."

Permission Denied

Most often visitors—subconsciously—may not want to know what worries their relative has about being laid up so long or how to take care of his family or his money problems or anything else. Deep inside, everyone has fears of something similar happening to oneself, and not talking about such things keeps them at bay. But determinedly sticking to trivialities and upbeat forecasts about how well everything is going for your relative denies permission for the expression of those fears—"trivial" or not—just when expression is most needed.

The "Invisible" Friend or Relative

Try to avoid talking in front of your injured friend or relative as if he or she isn't there: "We're feeling so much better today," or "We're not hungry right now," is an unconscious put-down of the person involved. Even saying, "She wants something to eat," is unnecessarily impersonal when you can perfectly well use a name. Personal names equal unique, living individuals with minds, feelings, and memories. Pronouns can stand for anyone—or a bureau, a tree, or a cow.

So, when you're with your buddy who fell off a roof or your mother who had hip surgery, say, "Joe would like something to eat," or "Mom is feeling better today." If Mom or Joe is able, better yet would be to ask, "Joe, didn't you say you wanted something to eat?" or "Mom, Jane called and wants to know how you're feeling today." Mom and Joe won't feel invisible.

Getting in Some Fun for Your Friend or Relative

Call in advance so that your friend or relative can anticipate your visit as well as "spiff up" a bit.

Immediately after a bad injury or unpleasant operation, listening or just being there is needed rather than entertaining. Later on, some of the following activities may be agreeable.

Suggest reading out loud a story or book that has been put aside for lack of energy. Frequently TV can be boring or tiring for a patient, but holding a book and concentrating on small black words is too demanding also. The sound of words, without the need to respond or even really listen can be comforting and soothing.

Audiocassettes and books on tape are also an alternative to TV and reading. Provide a player of some sort and get appropriate cassettes from your public library.

If your friend has a VCR, rent a movie or two for him or her, providing delivery and pickup service.

A big help can be to write thank-you notes for flowers and other gifts.

When the time is ripe, offer to take your pal or your parent on a jaunt of their choosing. Be sure to call ahead about accessibility — and if there is any possibility of getting a local handicapped parking permit, set about acquiring it now. See Chapter 15 for relevant suggestions.

Similarly, if your friend or family member has been part of a regular group such as one which meets to play cards or a sport, or a volunteer organization, or if he's in a close-knit office or carpool, try to get a group visit organized.

Fun for your friend or relative might be taking their children on an outing.

If recovery is going to be drawn-out, encourage participation in former activities in another way — such as coaching, consulting, editing, repairing, and restoring. Be searching for new outlets to suggest.

Balancing Your Life While Caring for Family

Patients get out of the hospital much sooner than they used to, even those who have had complicated joint replacements or plates screwed into shattered bones. Much more care is now given at home, and generally it imposes a brand-new role on those who are providing it.

Try to balance your needs and those of your injured wife, husband, parent, or offspring. Just because the patient's condition is temporary doesn't mean the recovery period is going to be over in a flash. Most likely it will be pretty long and drawn-out — the last visit to the physical therapist may be months down the road.

It's tricky, no doubt about it. But remember, if you become resentful, that it's easy to get angry, and after anger comes guilt, and then the whole family is affected negatively. Keep to established family routines if possible. Oversacrifice is not best — least of all for your gimpy/limpy family member or friend.

So, try to spend at least a little time each day in an activity unrelated to the person whom you are helping care for. If he or she really needs constant attention, see if a friend or relative will spell you for an hour once or twice a week. Try especially hard to maintain your own fitness routines: you need them now more than ever, both for health of body and of mind.

Helping Someone to Sit Up in Bed or Stand Up If Sitting

Positioning: Face the patient, noting which is the uninjured-side hand and arm.

Arm lock: Accomplish the arm lock by grasping the patient's arm underneath the elbow. His or her forearm will lie across your forearm, and he or she will grasp the inner portion of your elbow.

Hoist: Pull up slowly and steadily.

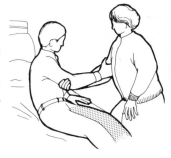

• • ●Word to the Wise: ARM CHOICE. This very helpful technique
works best if the hand you use is the same as the arm and hand of
the patient you are lifting. This makes better levering and means
that you reach your right hand under the patient's right elbow and
forearm—or left under left.

• • ●Word to the Wise: ESTABLISHING CRUTCHES. Avoid being
"tidy" and putting someone's crutches anyplace but right next to
him or her. Keep independence alive and well.

Helping Someone Stand Up Who Needs More Assistance

This provides more hoisting *oomph,* and may be useful for weaker or
overweight persons.

Positioning: Stand in front of the patient.

Arm lock: Slide your arms underneath the person's armpits and
clasp your hands behind his back.

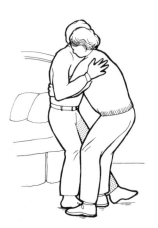

> *Note:* For added safety and lifting power, a "gait" or safety
> belt can be worn by the patient. Slide your arms around his
> waist and grab onto the safety belt rather than clothing—
> which might tear and give way. Such belts are found at
> medical-supply stores.

Optional leg "brace":   If extra levering is needed, place your knee
against the patient's good knee to help in straightening it to take
weight. Your arms will be circling the waist.

Hoist: Keep the person's weight forward as you aid him or her
to rise.

> *Caution:* Be sure your knees are bent to protect your back from strain.

Helping Someone Walk—With or Without Mobility Aids

When an individual is first using crutches or another aid, or is just beginning to use both legs again, you may want to be available to help. There are two methods to choose from depending upon the person and the situation.

Guarding from in front: Standing and backing up in front of the individual as they start out crutching or walking allows you to recognize anxiety, hesitation, or instability more easily. In addition, the patient's attention is focused more on reaching you than on the difficulties of the activity.

Guarding from behind: This positioning permits quicker aid if the individual is very tottery or uncertain. Stand on the involved side, about four to six inches behind. Point out a goal that the person should head for so that there is less awareness of you at the side and more concentration on performing the activity. A belt placed around the waist can provide a substantial boost in confidence for such persons. Gait belts, made specifically for this purpose, are recommended.

Assisting with Stairs

If your relative or friend is shaky, lacks strength or confidence, or is non-weight-bearing, it is prudent to be at hand the first few times he or she goes up or down stairs. See Chapter 8 for stair techniques.

Ascending: If weight can be placed on the injured leg, stand at the individual's side so he or she can use the handrail on one side, and you can be ready to aid on the other.

If crutches are being employed, stand behind the person with your feet in a stable "stride" position, one foot on the stair just below the patient and your other foot on the next stair down. Maintain that positioning as you follow.

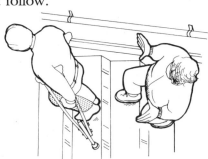

Descending: Aiding or being available for someone going downstairs is—unfortunately—a choice between two imperfect techniques. Positioning yourself in front can be a distraction and hindrance as the individual descends. Positioning behind or to the side makes it difficult to counteract gravity should there be a fall.

Positioning in front will place you in the stride mode, backing down the stairs as your friend or relative descends.

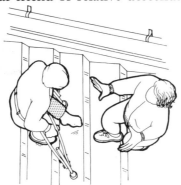

Positioning to the side—avoid being behind since your control will be minimal—means you should be prepared to grab the patient's waistband or a belt with one hand while placing the other under the armpit. Should helping in this hazardous fashion be a long-term situation, it is highly recommended that a gait belt be obtained for the patient.

Caution: In all situations involving stairs, ramps, etc., be sure your own center of gravity and base of support are firmly established and maintained in relation to the patient's weight and angle.

Aiding with stairs in a crowd: Congestion and hurrying people make for a dangerous situation for anyone moving hesitantly or using mobility aids. Follow behind your relative or friend to prevent him or her from being "run over" by the heedless masses.

Aiding Someone Using a Wheelchair

Some persons recovering from extensive surgery or accidents involving more than one leg, and those needing to conserve energy, will use wheelchairs to increase their independence. Read on for some words to the wise, and also see Chapter 6.

Attitude: Although the use of a wheelchair is probably temporarily in the situation of the relative or friend you're coping with, it's wise to be aware that persons in wheelchairs are often treated as if they were deaf, dumb, stupid, or ignorant. Don't let that virus spread in your vicinity.

Misperception: Besides being sane and healthy, most persons using wheelchairs are not paralyzed. Wheelchairs are more frequently used to conserve energy and for neurological conditions.

Ask first: It's always best to ask a person in a wheelchair if assistance is needed and, next, how to furnish it. Do not insist on helping.

Safety: It is essential that all helpers—family, friends, acquaintances, associates—are warned that brakes on a wheelchair must always be locked when the user is in the process of sitting or standing.

Footrest factor: Be aware that footrests and the feet on them will protrude from the chair.

Conversing with someone in a wheelchair: Sitting next to the wheelchair—rather than standing—is more considerate.

Wall whiteout: Try to avoid stopping the chair with your friend or relative facing a blank wall or similar area.

Neck cramp: Try to position the chair at the point where the rider can observe best, rather than the one from where you can see best—a common oversight. This spares the patient's having to look back over his shoulder—especially helpful in museums.

Entering an elevator: Press the button to lock the door open before pulling the wheelchair in backward.

Ramps: Ask your passenger to lean forward when going up a ramp to help control steering and prevent tipping over backward. Going down a ramp, tip the chair back onto its rear wheels or push it as usual while holding back on the handles to lessen speed.

Curbs: To mount a curb, approach and turn the wheelchair around. Tip the wheelchair back onto its large rear wheels by pressing the tipping lever with your foot and pulling back on the handles. Then tug it up over the curb, large wheels first. When the chair is fully on the sidewalk, lower the front so the small front wheels are in contact.

Going down a curb is normally done frontward (although the backward approach can work well too). With the front wheels near the curb, use the tipping lever to position the weight on the large rear wheels, and slowly roll and lower the chair over the edge. Then lower the front wheels to the ground, and off you both go.

Narrow spaces: Wheelchairs need less room for turning, when space is limited, if they are tilted back.

Recovery Wrap-Up: Last Thoughts and Thoughts to Last   18

"Recovery" is a devious word, one that can denote different stages on the road back to full mobility and fitness. One stage may be recuperation in the hospital, the next may be a certain amount of time unable to place weight on a leg, another may be learning to walk again, or the end of rehabilitation.

Ironically, renewed frustration and discouragement can be the result of arriving at the end of one of the stages of recovery. So much of oneself is invested in the various achievements of getting home, getting a cast off, and being able to bear weight again that the hard reality of the next stage is a tremendous shock. Euphoria flees fast.

The last medical visit—being *"cast off"* by the doctor—can produce not only anxiety but resentment and anger that things are not better than they are at that point. Understandably, the end of active professional care signals to some individuals that recovery has gone as far as is possible—resulting in tremendous disappointment and, occasionally, renunciation of long-term goals. It is important to remember that although medical treatment may be complete, recovery isn't.

The "Exceptional Patient" and the "Exceptional Athlete"

The patient with the best outlook for recovery is the one who is, as much as possible, self-reliant. (After all, you didn't get where you now are just because of doctors, operations, or pills.) The "exceptional patient" that Dr. Bernie Siegel singles out in *Love, Medicine and Miracles* is one that does not rely blindly on medical gods, but uses them as members of his or her team. Exceptional patients know to question decisions and realize that their ultimate progress will be due to satisfying themselves, not the man in white. They are aware that doctors' pronouncements tend to be dire and that people frequently do much—much!—better than predicted, and they are confident that they will

191

beat the odds that serious injury can impose. And if the consequences of injury cannot be entirely overcome, they do not, in Dr. Siegel's words, "cave in and allow it to disfigure their lives more than it should."

Dr. Siegel's reflection has particular relevance for athletes. At whatever level, an athlete's identification may well be with a sport and his or her prowess at it. Inability to ever play or perform again is devastating—not infrequently, the stages of an athlete's acceptance of permanent disability resemble those of facing terminal illness. Luckily there is a vast difference, and the opportunity remains to create anew where another might cave in. When the cheering stops it is halftime or time-out: what counts now is what one does during the rest of the game of life.

One of the Gang Again

Along with serious injury can come an outpouring of love and help in many forms. Without it the emotional and practical aspects of recovery are almost impossible to contemplate. But it is important to anticipate and prepare for the time that must inevitably come when you are no longer treated as a special project. See it not as abandonment but as a tribute to your progress. Progress means less and less attention and being treated like everyone else.

"How-are-you-doing?" inquiries will now likely be a part of normal social interaction and not really expressions of concern about or interest in your health. A fairly noncommital reply—"I'm fine. Thanks for asking."—covers the bases. Progress!

Estimated Time of Recovery: ETR

The stages of recovery may be easier to handle emotionally by calculating a *new* "ETR"—Estimated Time of Recovery—when you start walking without cast or brace. The old ETR, *surmised* (definitely the most apt designation) at the time of your accident or operation, is really no longer relevant. There can be all sorts of curves and potholes in the road before walking is permitted, but once that milestone is reached, Stage No. 1 is over and *another* ETR commences. Stage No. 2, rehabilitation, awaits.

Start a new countdown from the day you begin to walk again. Forget the last ETR—how many weeks before getting rid of the cast, or whatever it was. Adjust your mental sights to the fact that the muscles, tendons, and joints of your leg are just now being allowed to return to full use after a long layoff. Simply looking at the leg should warn you about the time that will be required, the hundreds of repetitive exercises still to be done, and the miles of walking or cycling or swimming to put in.

There's still a lot of determination and persistence to invest before those last two stages — rehabilitation and regaining fitness — are complete.

Communicating with Your Doctor

The two final stages of recovery are not easy. Rehabilitation is interminable, and regaining of fitness — cardiovascular, strength, and flexibility — is far down the road. It all will require more of what you've already been through.

To start with — since physicians vary in communication skills — informing yourself can take persistence in ferreting out important details relating to your getting back in shape. Surveys indicate that most doctors underestimate their patients' desire for information from the very beginning and, even worse, are poor at giving clear instructions. Don't be put off by the subtle sense of hurry on your doctor's part or possibly your own mixed feelings that your questions are trivial or not worth bothering the doctor with. You are paying for expertise — and no doubt it's a lot you're paying — so get the product you're buying.

If possible, come in with a written list of questions. Be specific. "May I start Nautilus workouts again?" and "Are there any machines I should avoid?" "How about cycling, Stairmaster, NordicTrack?" — or whatever your particular passion is. "Should I ice after exercise?" "Is pain to be expected, and if so, do I work through it or back off?" No doubt you will *not* think of everything in advance — in that case, persist some more and call. The nurse will get answers for you, or your doctor will return the call.

The next move is to write down what your doctor tells you, either after you leave his office or right there. If the latter, read it back for verification. The doctor gets to reconsider and add to what he or she has told you, and you know you have the correct information — both for verification and referral if needed later on. If you have phone consultations with your doctor, jot down your questions before making the call and make notes of the instructions as well. Date and hold on to these records. They can help you keep track of symptoms that may be important for future evaluation.

Rehabilitation and Physical Therapy

Rehabilitation, Stage No. 2 of recovery, usually commences soon after injury or surgery but doesn't get really rolling until you're allowed to put weight on your injured leg again. Estimated Time of Recovery No. 2 now begins.

The goal of rehabilitation used to be just to make people functional in ordinary living skills; now the goal is getting you back to your highest possible level of activity no matter what it is. This is accomplished through exercises you do by yourself at home and increasingly through treatments and exercises prescribed by your doctor and administered by professional physical therapists.

Physical therapy speeds recovery immeasurably. A doctor's prescription is required; if your doc is one of the few who doesn't routinely recommend rehabilitative therapy, ask for a prescription and let the PT experts show you their magic. Their knowledge of appropriate and recovery-hastening exercise far exceeds that of the majority of "white coats." Luckily, most physicans know it. After an initial evaluation, physical-therapy sessions last from 30 to 60 minutes apiece and are scheduled two or three days a week—generally three to start with.

Learning to do your PT exercises correctly is an essential part of physical therapy and the rehabilitation of your leg. Keep in mind that although your injury may have been to a foot, a non-weight-bearing regimen, wearing a cast, and abnormal gait (limping) affect the *entire* leg—all the way to the hip and often to the back as well. Rehabilitation should focus on the whole picture.

Physical therapists are also able to evaluate whether your discomfort in various exercises is appropriate for the injury and stage of recovery—a great help and source of relief and confidence. "Let pain be your guide" is altogether too ambiguous—inspiring too much caution in some individuals while others work their way through pain to their detriment. Nice to have someone else deciding those things.

Rehabilitation frequently does not end with the last of your professional therapy sessions. Exercises performed at home may continue for months, and—particularly in cases of knee injury—may need to be done permanently. It's an awful prospect to be "sentenced to quadriceps exercise for life," and a majority of people give up eventually. However, you need not be one of them if you alternate in doing just two—but *at least one!*—of your prescribed exercises each day. (Visually cue yourself by stationing your weights where you can't fail to be reminded by them—on your bed, for instance.) Doing that one exercise is better, much better, than doing none at all, and your leg muscles may stay strong enough and balanced enough to forestall another injury. "Hate it"—but heed the advice.

Getting Back to Active Pastimes

Returning to fitness is Stage No. 3, the final goal. Usually when the consequences of injury or operation are estimated, the time it will take to regain former levels of fitness, strength, and flexibility is entirely overlooked in the calculation. Unless you are a professional athlete, doctors rarely consider return to good fitness as your ETR—and if they do, then the ETR they suggest is likely to be when you can *start* an energetic activity again rather than when you will be fully in shape and fully retrained to play or do the activity as you did before injury. That requires more weeks—most likely several months—at the very least.

So on top of time-out for an injury or surgery are the time-outs for rehabilitation therapy and for building your important body systems back up again to the point where they're ready for your own particular lifestyle. If that is no more demanding than walking from your car to your office, you won't have so far to go, and the prospect won't be so frustrating. But if it's a sport or sports you plan to return to—whether as a full-time athlete or a weekend warrior—pacing yourself now is of crucial importance.

Ideally you have had fitness in mind throughout your recovery and have been working on aspects of it all along, as suggested in Chapters 3 and 4. But as recommended previously, if you're just starting to work on strength and endurance, proceed as in early-season sunbathing: start with 15 minutes, and work up gradually. Follow the "rules of road" outlined in Chapter 2: green light and proceed with the activity if there is no pain or other symptom of stress; yellow light and caution if there are moderate symptoms which do not increase or worsen with continuation of the activity; red light, stop and consult your therapist or doctor, if symptoms worsen.

Rehabilitation can be discouraging, because new pains seem to crop up without cause or warning. Evaluate them according to the "rules of the road," above, while also realizing complaints are to be expected as muscles, joints, tendons, ligaments, and systems throughout the body come out of hibernation. Inactivity lulls one into thinking the body must be great—and grateful for all the rest. False. Stay smart and stay slow on getting back. Most pains will prove to be temporary; try backing off the discomfort-producing activity for a few days or weeks and then giving it another whirl.

Be particularly careful if you participate in sports that involve running (especially on hard surfaces). Although your muscle rebuilding may be complete, bone is produced or replaced more slowly than muscle tissue and needs extra time of gradual stressing to get stronger. Train too hard—or too hard too soon—or too fast, and your muscles may accommodate but your bones may not. Stress fractures are the result.

Accentuating the Positive

At any stage of recovery, it is worthwhile to consider whether you can create out of this difficult interlude in your life something positive both for yourself and for others. Many persons' lives are unalterably changed when injury or illness—limited or long-term—forcibly requires restructuring and rethinking of priorities. Physical pain, helplessness, dependency, new and unimagined shocks of all kinds, lead to a treasuring and clasping of many facets of life previously taken for granted.

Often this period is a catalyst in understanding and empathizing with the suffering of others for the first time in a person's life. For some comes the realization that in truth most of us are only *temporarily* able-bodied persons. Joining the disabled minority not only can happen at any time but is pretty likely to happen anyway if one lives long enough. Creating something, helping some person or cause, or supporting organizations that do, can be a meaningful reflection of a new-found awareness and gratitude for what one has.

The Void Doesn't Last Long

Amazingly, reaching the finish line on that road to recovery can be unsettling in itself—particularly if it's been a long one, perhaps with several operations or repeated reinjury. Working to come back can dominate one's life. The requirements of recovery—rehabilitation, therapy, exercise, stretching, strengthening, walking skills and walking strength, returning to high-performance fitness and high-performance skills if a professional athlete—become one's existence.

Strangely, when you have achieved or mostly achieved what all the struggle has been about, something seems to be *missing:* that never-ending battle! It's wonderful—unbelievable—to have it finally finished, yet the domination can have been so complete that it is now awkward no longer to be in the shoes of the struggler, no longer to have the full-time job of recovery, of getting back. Ironically, there's a void.

It's a void to be filled—but it never remains empty for very long.

Although physical limitations may now be a fact of life, later on a realization may come that you are finally *fully* recovered — that your overall capabilities, both mental and physical, are once more in sync and at full energy again. Work, chores, responsibilities, and extracurricular activities — despite limitations — no longer seem so monumental. Acceptance achieves this balance.

Acceptance of physical limitations is possible because so much is left; because you know where you are on that "ladder of suffering" that exists for everyone. A balance has been reached between goals desired and goals achieved.

19   Resource Information

The first part of this chapter is an alphabetical list of the individual items of equipment mentioned in the body of the text. Following the description of an item there is a number—or numbers—referring to the supply companies listed on pages 201-02 that offer this equipment. (The catalogs from these companies contain other items in addition to the ones listed here which you might find helpful.) The second part is a listing of exercise videos and an audiocassette, all of which are critiqued for level of difficulty, safety, and enjoyment. The final section contains some suggestions aimed at making travel and recreation easier.

The inclusion of publications, videotapes, equipment manufacturers, travel companies, and agencies or organizations of any kind do not constitute an endorsement by the author or publisher, but are provided solely for your information and convenience. Unfortunately, the information provided here cannot be guaranteed to be up-to-date, nor may all the products necessarily be available.

EQUIPMENT

Ankle Weights: These wrap-around weights are made of heavy-duty plastic filled with water to indicated levels and held on by Velcro straps. There are two sizes which range from one to three pounds or four to six pounds depending upon the amount of water added. An ingenious solution to the problem of quadriceps maintenance, as they are truly portable—weighing nothing and packing flat. The main drawback is that the water-entry closures are difficult to operate. (5)

Aqua Jogger: The Aqua Jogger is a water exercise belt used for training and rehabilitation after injury by athletes of all kinds. Frequently, fitness is not only maintained but actually improved. It is easy to adjust, does not restrict breathing, provides an excellent, jolt-free cardiovascular workout and comes with directions for use. (7)

Bathtub or shower benches or chairs: Polyethylene or vinyl-coated seats are very helpful aids to getting in and out of the tub for the mobility-impaired. One model, the "Easy-Enter" transfer bench, has a back rest that can be reversed from one side to the opposite side, depending on leg involvement. The height is adjustable.(4, 6, 10, 14)

Bathtub safety rail: Easily installed handgrips to enhance stability when getting in and out of a tub. (4, 14)

Beanbag lap desk: A portable, lap-conforming desk. (4)

Bed tray: This tray doesn't have side compartments but does have legs that fold flat for storage. (4)

Bedpan, fracture: A smaller, thinner bedpan which is more easily positioned under the buttocks. Having one at hand lends assurance when getting to the bathroom is difficult, and for females serves the same needs as a male urinal. (4)

Bedside caddy: A storage pocket that tucks in between the mattress and bedspring for easy access to frequently used or misplaced items. (4)

Cane: A standard mobility aid available in various shapes and materials. See Chapter 6 for more on the different models available. (14)

Cane clip: A clip that will attach the cane to a counter or table top to keep it close at hand. (4, 10)

Cane, folding: A 36″ cane that reduces to a size that will fit into your pocket or tote bag. (4)

Cane tip, high-tech: See under "Crutch tips, high-tech," below.

Cane tip, "ice pick": These are specialized tips for wintertime use on snow and ice. They enhance safety in such conditions although, in general, travel on ice or snow is not recommended for those with compromised stability. (6, 10, 13)

Cast protectors: Surgical-grade latex cast protectors for bathing which slip on like a sock, seal snugly at the top, and can be reused indefinitely. Shapes for feet, ankles, half-leg, and full-leg casts, and sizes for men, women, and children. (9)

Crutch tips, high-tech: These tips have a unique, two-piece steel ball-and-socket joint that enables the crutch or cane to maintain full contact with the ground at all times for extra holding ability and maneuverability. The bottom face has small projections for greater security. (6, 10, 13)

Crutches: Standard mobility aids available in several models. See Chapter 5 for details.

Cuff weights: Weighted leather straps that wrap around either ankles or wrists and fasten with Velcro; available in graduated weights. (10)

Driving Aids: Adaptive equipment for cars—quite reasonable in price—that will make driving possible for almost anybody. Persons with right-leg injury can get a left-foot accelerator. If both legs are involved, hand-operated brake and throttle controls are available and easily installed. The adaptive equipment does not prevent normal operation of the car. Drivers new to the adaptive equipment must be careful to keep clear of the regular brake and accelerator pedals. (8)

Elastic shoelaces: These laces are threaded into tie shoes, and because of their stretch one's foot can be slid into or removed from the shoe without needing to tie or untie it. (10)

Gait or walker belts: A belt designed to go around the waist of a patient who is overweight or unusually weak or fearful. The belt is gripped by the person who is aiding, either helping the patient to rise or to provide stability and confidence in employment of mobility aids. Use of such a belt is preferable to holding on to a patient's clothes or personal belt, which may give way. (1)

Hospital-style, over-bed table: An adjustable-height table on casters the base of which slides under the bed. It can be folded for storage. (2, 6, 10, 14)

Lap tray: A tray to use in bed that sits on the lap. (2, 6, 10, 14)

Leg elevator: A shaped piece of foam rubber that can be used instead of a pillow or pillows to elevate a leg. (1)

Pants, zipper: Pants with full-length side zippers that can be unzipped at both the waist and ankle; extremely practical and easy to use. (11, 12)

Reachers: Various reachers from the simplest to deluxe, any of which will prevent a lot of energy-depleting retrievals. (1, 4, 10)

Reclining lounge chair: A chair that provides an easy and extremely comfortable method of leg elevation, without the risk of back problems or the aggravation of pillows which slip and slide. The drawbacks are the space required for the chair as well as the cost. (14)

Shoe aids: Such aids are specialized reachers that help in getting a shoe on or off. They are useful for persons with full-length casts or limitations due to arthritis. (6, 10)

Shower heads, hand-held: Fixtures available that can be permanently installed or which attach to a faucet with no hardware required. A five foot plastic hose makes washing and shampooing easy, especially when using a bathtub or shower bench. (4, 14)

Sock, stocking aids: Specialized reachers like shoe aids; see above.

Surgical tubing: Thin, stretchable, rubber tubing which provides resistance and is used in rehabilitation exercises. (1, 10)

Theraband: Stretchable rubber straps or bands in different widths which provide resistance and are used in rehabilitation exercises. (1, 10)

Toilet safety rail: An easily and extremely helpful installed aid for persons with sitting, standing, or balance difficulties. It mounts between the toilet seat and bowl and requires no wall or floor connections. (4, 10, 14)

Toilet seat, elevated: This seat adds almost six inches to the height of a standard toilet; another model is adjustable. Fits all toilet bowls. (1, 4, 6, 10, 14)

Tongs: Extra long cooking implement to ensure safe reaching over front burners of a stove for those using crutches, walkers, or wheelchairs. They can also be used for retrievals. (4)

Walker: A standard mobility aid available in several models and sizes. See Chapter 6 for details.

Walker bag: A tote bag for a walker or wheelchair with velcro straps for attachment and two large pockets. (4, 6, 10)

Walker basket: A basket that attaches to the front of a walker and includes a holder for a soft drink can or cup. (4, 14)

Wet Vest: The Wet Vest is a body-enveloping water exercise garment that ressembles a vest with a crotch piece added for fitting purposes. Its uses are similar to the Aqua Jogger, but fitting and putting on the vest are more complicated. (3)

Wheelchair: A standard mobility aid available in many models and sizes suitable for all types of injuries. See Chapter 6 for details.

Wheelchair tray: Attaches to the armrests of the wheelchair and is used for dining, work, and recreational needs. (6, 10, 14)

Suppliers:

1. **Alimed, Inc.**
   297 High Street
   Dedham, MA 02026-2839
   800-225-2610

2. **The Alsto Company**
   P.O. Box 1267
   Galesburg, IL 61401
   800-447-0048

3. **Bioenergetics, Inc.**
   5074 Shelby Drive
   Birmingham, AL 35243
   800-433-2627

4. **Bruce Medical Supply**
   411 Waverly Oaks Road
   P.O. Box 9166
   Waltham, MA 02254-9166
   800-225-8446

5. **Caef, Inc.**
   11705 Cypress Park
   Tampa, FL 33624

6. **Comfortably Yours**
   61 West Hunter Ave.
   Maywood, NJ 07607-1005
   201-368-0400

7. **Excel Sports Science, Inc.**
   P.O. Box 5612
   Eugene, Oregon 97405
   800-922-9544

8. **Gresham Driving Aids**
   Box 405 A
   30800 Wixom Road
   Wixom, MI 48096
   800-521-8930; 313-624-1533

9. **Little and Co.**
   Grand Junction, CO 81505
   800-854-3155

10. **Maddak, Inc.**
    Pequannock, NJ 07440
    201-628-7600

11. **Patagonia**
    1609 W. Babcock St.
    P.O. Box 8900
    Bozeman, MT 59715-2046
    800-638-6364

12. **REI**
    P.O. Box 88125
    Seattle, WA
    800-426-4840

13. **The Rehab Shoppe**
    3957 Mayfield Road
    Cleveland, OH 44121
    800-321-0595; 216-382-9700

14. **Sears Health Care Catalog**
    Sears Roebuck Co.
    P.O. Box 780593
    Wichita, KS 67278
    800-366-3000
    or P.O. Box 27900
    San Antonio, TX 78227
    800-366-3000
    (west of the Mississippi)

AUDIO AND VIDEO EXERCISE PRODUCTS

Having someone lead you in a safe and energetic exercise routine without leaving your room has advantages. It's easy, it's motivating, and the fact that the persons demonstrating the routines are generally gorgeous — with a few handsomes thrown in — isn't so bad either. Music varies but is generally a great addition. Videos are included here for every stage and every age.

Don't exclude a video because it was designed for a disability that you don't have. The exercises and how they are done are what count. The evaluations will help you choose which one is right for you at your particular stage of recovery — after first getting permission from your physician or therapist. The listing goes, in general, from the least amount of leg involvement to the greatest.

Janet Reed's *Wheelchair Workout* is an audiocassette for people in an early stage of recovery who have no access to a TV, dislike television, or wish to exercise where none is available. It provides an excellent upper-body workout with an extensive warmup that leads into accelerated exercise. The verbal instructions are clear and easily followed, and Reed's voice imparts calm and warm reinforcement. Write to: 12275 Greenleaf Ave., Potomac, MD 20854.

Karen Wilson's *Sit and Be Fit*

As this video is designed for persons in wheelchairs, the emphasis is on an upper-body workout—and a good one it is. You'll know you got real exercise, even though the video doesn't include the walking or running you wish you could do. Karen Wilson is perfect as the demonstrator, achieving the right mix of no-nonsense and encouragement. Sit and Be Fit, 10201 North 58th Place, Scottsdale, AZ 85253.

Slabo Productions' *Keep Fit While You Sit*

A video which stands out for its excellent variety in warmup, stretching, and isometric exercise as well as the concluding fast-paced upper-body workout. The music is bouncy and rhythmic; this tape comes off as a fun way to exercise your above-waist area while the below-waist area relaxes. Write to: Slabo Productions, 1057 South Crescent Heights Boulevard, Los Angeles, CA 90035.

Richard Simmons' *Reach for Fitness: A Complete Fitness Program for the Physically Challenged*

A video designed for those in wheelchairs but useful for anyone unable to walk or do meaningful exercise requiring use of the legs. This routine, done sitting, is a vigorous, non-stop action of arms, hands, torso, etc. After a preliminary pitch for good nutrition and avoidance of fat, the presentation is perky—almost too perky—and comes off as a bit too "nobly uplifting" for someone dealing with a permanent disability. However, it's the exercise that counts and this is suitable for the earliest stages of recovery. Warner Home Video, 4000 Warner Boulevard, Burbank, CA 91522 (or your video store).

National Multiple Sclerosis Society's *The MS Wheelchair Workout* and *The MS Workout*

The first of these workouts is suitable for anyone who is still unable to walk following leg surgery or injury. The second MS video incorporates standing and lying down exercises as well as stretches appropriate for persons in the beginning and middle stages of recovery from lower leg injury. *The MS Workout* is demonstrated by Jimmy Huega, former U.S. Ski Team member and Olympic medalist. Contact the Multiple Sclerosis Society, 205 E. 42nd Street, New York, NY 212-986-3240.

Maura Casey's *Walkerobics*

Created to increase and maintain the endurance of the no-longer-so-young set, the video has both sitting and standing exercise routines. The standing exercises, done while holding on to a walker or chair, are presented nonstop and constitute a good lower-extremity workout after extended inactivity. The music helps keep you revved up. Casey-Dipery Enterprises, P.O. Box 723, Butler, NJ 07407.

Jane Fonda's *Workout with Weights* gives very good demonstrations of some of the exercises included in the fitness chapters of *Getting Back on Your Feet* — as well as lots more. There are beginners' and advanced levels, good warmups, and stretches throughout are included. With frequent reminders, Fonda emphasizes paying attention to proper form, as well as pointing out less demanding ways of doing each exercise. The music is energizing, and the exercises are nonstop — you are encouraged to "opt out" when you need to. This tape is suitable for any stage of recovery through selection and elimination of inappropriate or unachievable exercises. This and the following Fonda videos are available from Warner Home Video, 4000 Warner Blvd, Burbank, CA 91522 (or your video store).

New Workout, divided into beginner and advanced ability levels, is best used for achieving fitness near the end of your recovery period, when both legs are on "green light." This is active, speedy, nonstop fun, with great music and pizzaz. Stretches are emphasized and extensive in both the beginner and advanced portions.

Easy Going Workout is also called "Prime Time Workout," and starts off with toning of the legs, arms, shoulders, and waist through stretching followed by a series of leg exercises performed while holding on to a chair for support which will help with your range of motion. This warmup is suitable for an advanced stage of recovery; the section which follows — requiring vigorous leg involvement — will need to be saved for the day when both legs are back in top shape. Good music makes this a cheerful workout.

Low Impact Aerobic Workout is a full-body workout that starts with warmup, gradually increases pace, and ends with cool-down and stretches. One foot is on the floor at all times during the leg exercises. This is a controlled but nonstop session suitable for a stage of advanced recovery. The music is a catchy mix of styles.

Sports Aid is a well-organized and presented first-aid video about the most common injuries to various parts of the body. Dr. James Garrick, a noted sports medicine/orthopaedic doctor at San Francisco's Saint Francis Memorial Hospital, discusses each type of injury thoroughly, explaining what has occurred and what symptoms would indicate seeing a doctor. Fonda, along with props and a willing model, demonstrates what one does at home if a serious injury is not indicated. Because of the visual demonstrations, this is a good addition to one's first-aid center.

RECREATION AND TRAVEL

ParaTransit System, New York City and other metropolises: "Access-A-Ride" is a city-wide, door-to-door, advance-reservation, shared-ride transportation service. It requires customers to be certified as "transportation-disabled," which includes inability to stand alone without crutches, canes, walkers, braces, or other assistance. Temporary disablement status (three months minimum) is possible if certified by an M.D. or licensed physical therapist. Trips are either demand-responsive for random needs or by subscription for regularly recurring rides to the same destination. Funding constraints place limits on this service. Similar systems exist in other large cities.

Train travel: Write to Amtrak, National Railroad Passenger Corp., Public Affairs Office, 400 North Capital Street, N.W., Washington, DC 20001, or call 800-872-7245, for *Access Amtrak: A Guide for Elderly and Handicapped Travelers*, which will help you on questions of accessibility and services. Train travel with Amtrak is a good choice for a person with mobility problems. Employees get special training in assistance, and meals can be requested to be brought to you if walking in a moving train is risky.

Car rental: For the determined person who has both legs out of commission, cars with hand controls can be rented if advance notice is given. Since two-legged disability means you will also be using a wheelchair, cars with two doors—rather than four—are preferable because of the extra room between the driver's seat and the back seat where the chair gets stowed. Cars with hand controls are likely to be available only in large cities.

Avis: 800-331-1212, domestic reservations
800-331-2112, international reservations
(3 weeks advance notice)

Hertz: 800-654-3131 (10 days advance notice)

National: 800-328-4567 (3 days advance notice)

Cruises: If you had a great vacation planned and have to give it up because of a broken leg, a knee reconstruction, or a sprained ankle, substituting a cruise is a wonderful option. Many, many ships have been adapted with the mobility-impaired in mind, which — at the moment — means you too. For information on such ships, check with a knowledgeable travel agent (see listing below) and/ or: Cruise Lines International, 500 Fifth Avenue, Suite 1407, New York, NY 10110. Ask for their *Cruise Guide for the Wheelchair Traveler* and *Cruising*, which answer general-interest questions. They also have a chart listing 87 ships with the features offered mobility-impaired passengers, obtained by sending $1 and a stamped, self-addressed envelope.

Travel Agencies with special expertise and special tours: The tours organized by these agencies — both domestic and overseas — are helpful not only for persons using any type of mobility aid but also for those who are slowed down for other causes. A slower pace is taken for granted, elevators are used that are not available to the general public, and other energy-conserving services are provided. Such specialized agencies can save you a lot of time in arranging details of travel when an accident has suddenly intruded on your life.

Directions Unlimited
720 North Bedford Road
Bedford Hills, New York 10507
800-533-5343; 914-241-1700

Flying Wheels Travel
P.O. Box 382
143 West Bridge Street
Owatonna, MN 55060
800-533-0363; 507-451-5005

Evergreen Travel Service
19505 44th Avenue West
Lynnwood, WA 98036
800-435-2288; 206-776-1184

Accessibility of national parks: A marvelous guide, *Access America: An Atlas of the National Parks for Visitors with Disabilities* details all sorts of essential information — and would be helpful for *anyone* scouting a trip to one of our popular national parks, both east and west. The large format makes it a joy to use, and the design — focusing on ease of use by readers with many types of disabilities- —will also be cherished by the public at large. The atlas has big print for readers with visual difficulties, easily handled paper and spiral binding for those having motor disabilities, and a semihard cover to reduce weight.

For the mobility-impaired, the atlas evaluates access to parking, visitor centers, exhibits, amphitheaters, restrooms, campground sites, ramp gradients, pathway and door widths, as well as selected eating, lodging, and supplies concessionaires.

Diagrams are provided of visitor centers and climate and weather information is noted. Best of all are the 300 large, multicolored maps, drawings, and full-color photos. There is a 25 percent discount for individuals purchasing the atlas for their own use. Also check libraries. Booklets for individual parks are in the works. Contact: Northern Cartographic, Box 133, Burlington, VT 05402, or call 802-655-4321.

Another way to check accessibility of parks is to contact the park yourself. Get a listing from the Department of Interior, National Park Service, P.O. Box 37127, Washington, DC, 20013-7127. The Interior Department also publishes *Access National Parks*, a booklet that can be obtained by writing the Superintendent of Documents, U.S. Government Printing Office, Washington, DC, 20402.

Index

Getting Back on Your Feet was designed
by Sally Harris/Summer Hill Books,
typeset in Galliard by the Dartmouth Printing Company,
and printed on Lynx Opaque Vellum, an acid-free paper,
by Princeton University Press.